Passing On

Inheritance, once the preserve of the propertied upper classes, has become a much more common experience. Many more people now have something of material value to bequeath when they die, mainly because of the spread of home ownership during the second half of the twentieth century. *Passing On* examines what these changes can tell us about kinship in England, through a study of how contemporary families handle inheritance.

Based on the findings of a major research project into inheritance and kinship, *Passing On* examines how property and possessions are transmitted, 'who gets what' and the meaning this has for individuals and families. The authors argue that we should understand English kinship as a set of relational practices which are flexible and variable, rather than as a rigid structure or system. Inheritance is characterised more by symbolic practices and moral reasoning than by materialism.

Of interest to lecturers and students of sociology, anthropology, social policy, law and gender studies, *Passing On* is also of considerable relevance to those seeking to understand changing forms of kinship and ownership, especially researchers, policy makers and legal practitioners.

Janet Finch is Vice Chancellor of Keele University. **Jennifer Mason** is Senior Lecturer in Sociology and Deputy Director of the Centre for Research on Family, Kinship and Childhood at the University of Leeds.

Passing On

Kinship and inheritance in England

Janet Finch and Jennifer Mason

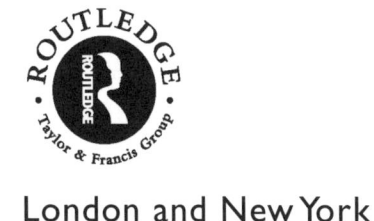

London and New York

First published 2000
by Routledge
11 New Fetter Lane, London EC4P 4EE

Simultaneously published in the USA and Canada
by Routledge
29 West 35th Street, New York, NY 10001

Routledge is an imprint of the Taylor & Francis Group

© 2000 Janet Finch and Jennifer Mason

Typeset in Sabon by Taylor & Francis Books Ltd
Printed and bound in Great Britain by Biddles Ltd,
Guildford and King's Lynn

All rights reserved. No part of this book may be reprinted or
reproduced or utilised in any form or by any electronic, mechanical,
or other means, now known or hereafter invented, including
photocopying and recording, or in any information storage or
retrieval system, without permission in writing from the publishers.

British Library Cataloguing in Publication Data
A catalogue record for this book is available from the British Library

Library of Congress Cataloging in Publication Data
Finch, Janet.
Passing on : kinship and inheritance in England / Janet Finch
and Jennifer Mason.
Includes bibliographical references and index.
1. Land tenure–Social aspects–England.
2. Inheritance and succession–Social aspects–England.
3. Kinship–England. 4. Family–England.
I. Mason, Jennifer, 1958– II. Title.
HD606 .F56 2000
333.3'23'0942–dc21   00-042476

ISBN 1–857–28276–0 (hbk)
ISBN 1–857–28277–9 (pbk)

Contents

Acknowledgements vi

1 Making connections: kinship and inheritance 1

2 Questions of complexity: a case study 25

3 Transmissions and divisions 62

4 Moral dilemmas 88

5 Questions of ownership 111

6 Symbolism 139

7 Drawing conclusions: kinship and inheritance 162

Appendix A: Methodology 183
Bibliography 189
Index 193

Acknowledgements

We would like to acknowledge with gratitude the support of the Economic and Social Research Council, which funded the research project on which this book is based (R00232035). As well as the authors, the research team included Lynn Hayes, Lorraine Wallis and Judith Masson, who have co-authored other publications arising from this research. We are very grateful for their involvement and their very significant contributions to the project. Janet Hartley, Pam Holme, Nichola Hetherington and Sandra Irving were secretaries on the project at different stages, and we are grateful to each of them for their efficiency, enthusiasm and sheer hard work. Others helped at various times with research assistance, and we would like to express our thanks in this respect to Hilary Conway, Jennifer Flowerdew and Diane Nutt. Finally, we would like to thank all our interviewees for so generously sharing their experiences of inheritance and kinship with us.

Chapter 1

Making connections
Kinship and inheritance

Introduction

What will happen to your possessions, and your assets if you have any, when you die? Does this concern you? Have you ever inherited anything? What did you do with it? What does it mean to you? Do you think there is a proper way for these matters to be worked out and resolved? To what extent are all these issues tied up with your own family relationships, and with your feelings about and connections with specific individuals?

These are the kinds of questions with which this book is concerned. It is an exploration of the relationships between inheritance of property and kinship, as expressed in people's hopes and fears, plans and strategies, actions and reasoning in relation to the role of inheritance in their own lives.

Inheritance of property is a topic relatively little studied and in one sense is the focus of this book. In later chapters, we shall present data from a set of empirical studies on how families handle the transmission of property after someone has died or in anticipation of death. Our focus is on inheritance and *material* property – personal possessions, objects, commodities, assets – both valuable and not.

Property inheritance is an intrinsically interesting topic in the contemporary English context because it involves many more people than in previous generations. The critical change here is the increasing rate of home ownership. Whereas in previous generations many people had little of material value to pass on to succeeding generations, the ownership of a house means that there is something valuable to bequeath. By 1997, 68 per cent of homes in the UK were owner-occupied. This is double the number of thirty years previously. Although the percentages are even higher for the most affluent sections of society, the fastest *rates* of growth have been among manual occupational groups. By 1996, three-quarters of skilled manual workers owned their own home, whereas the figure had been only half in 1981. Over the same period, the proportion of semi-skilled and unskilled manual workers who owned their own homes doubled (although the proportion currently owning homes remains lower than for other social groups) (Office for National Statistics 1999: 168–9).

The general picture is clear. Home ownership is no longer for just the relatively affluent. It is now a normal experience for 'ordinary families' (by which we mean those who have not owned considerable wealth or land over several generations), and across the full range of occupational groups. The corollary is that inheritance is now relevant to the majority of families. Under the Conservative governments of the 1980s and 1990s, this connection between home ownership and inheritance was made a political virtue as a way of binding citizens into the economic order of a property-owning democracy. Most famously John Major, when prime minister, spoke of a vision of Britain in which more and more families would be able to see 'wealth trickling down the generations'. In this vision, both families and society are bound together through the mechanism of inheritance.

However, in an important sense the central focus of this book is not inheritance but kinship. In examining how families handle inheritance, our focus is not so much on the property as on the relationships. When we look carefully, we can see that kin relationships are not simply the backdrop against which dramas concerned with inheritance get played out. They are themselves the real point. Individuals, we shall argue, do not simply make use of their relationships to acquire items of property, whether large or small. Rather, in the process of handling the transmission of property, the character and quality of those relationships is revealed, understood and remade by the participants.

In seeing inheritance as a process that *constitutes* families, not simply reflects them, we are following much of the classical anthropological and historical literature on kinship. Of course there are important political and cultural differences between societies, which make generalisations impossible. Nonetheless, it is a commonplace finding in much of this literature that property expresses and symbolises both the boundaries of a kinship group and the power structure within those boundaries. Its transmission following the death of one member is a critical process in adapting the group to new circumstances. For example, the distinguished anthropologist Jack Goody, writing of inheritance in Western European societies between 1200 and 1800, describes inheritance as 'the means by which the reproduction of the social system is carried out' (Goody 1976: 1). This underlines just how fundamental is the passing on of property to the constitution of the society itself. The 'reproduction of the social system' in this way is accomplished by means of consolidating family relationships in particular forms and shapes across generations. A similar view of the significance of kinship and inheritance is found in all the classical work in this historical-anthropological tradition (see, for example, Goody *et al.* 1976; Segalen 1986; Smith 1984).

Although we shall draw a number of insights from this literature, its relevance to the contemporary English context is limited for one important reason, namely the legal structure under which property is transmitted. The key point here is testamentary freedom. Within the English legal framework, each of us has a right to decide how to dispose of our property after we die, as well as during life. Although there are some restrictions upon this, especially where a testator has failed to leave property to people who were economically dependent upon him or her, this is very much at the margins of a system that otherwise privileges the choice of the individual. This approach to property transmission contrasts markedly with those legal jurisdictions, covering much of Europe, where a testator is required to bequeath to named individuals (for example, each child) in specified proportions (for more detailed discussion of these points, and their relevance to kinship, see Finch *et al.* 1996: chapter 2).

The very open-ended nature of the law of property transmission means that, in the English context, inheritance can give insights into kinship in a way that is impossible under those legal jurisdictions that give individuals less freedom of choice and where a testator is required to leave property to named individuals. The fact that English testators can *choose* how they dispose of their property means that the scene is set for using property transmission to constitute relationships in an active and meaningful way. As we shall argue below, the English kinship 'structure' itself also makes this possible.

When we put these two factors together, we can see that viewing kinship through the set of lenses provided by inheritance offers a rich set of possibilities for understanding the nature of contemporary kinship. It is particularly illuminating in a situation where many people are having to confront issues of inheritance for the first time within their own family contexts, since in previous generations there would have been nothing valuable to bequeath. Active engagement is required here, potentially making visible assumptions about who 'counts' sufficiently to receive a share of property.

Throughout the book we use both the terms 'family' and 'kinship'. We intend the use of these terms to be generous rather than restrictive, not least because we see the nature and meaning of the families and kinship that are constructed through inheritance as matters for investigation, as open questions that we can go some way towards addressing. We agree wholeheartedly with Smart and Neale when they say that 'it is still impossible to talk innocently of *the* family. There is too much diversity in family life to use such a homogenizing concept' (1999: 21).

In preference, they draw on Morgan's concept of 'family practices', which are 'those relationships and activities that are constructed as being to do with family matters', both by the actors involved and through 'processes of historical construction' (Morgan 1996: 192). This is significant for our study, because the term 'family' does have a meaning, although not a uniform one, for people in everyday life, and it also has meanings that have been activated historically through, most notably for our concerns, English inheritance law and legal discourses. In a strong sense, inheritance is 'constructed as being to do with family matters', so we have retained the term 'family' in this book, but we emphasise again that its use is intended to be generous and is certainly not innocent.

The term 'kinship' has less everyday or discursive resonance. We use it nevertheless partly because we wish to engage with intellectual debates about the nature and constitution of kinship but also because there is a sense in which 'kinship' is increasingly being claimed as a term that can express something wider, or more diverse, than 'family' in its most restrictive sense (see, for example, Weeks *et al.* 1999). As we have pointed out, this book is essentially about kinship: what that is, how it operates, where it is located and what it means are, for the present, open questions to which we shall return in the light of our data.

The contemporary significance of kinship

Family and kin relationships are a feature of all our lives, except in unusual circumstances. The sociological study of these relationships therefore possibly needs little justification. However, there are particular reasons for highlighting their significance at the present time which have informed our own thinking and with which we will engage in the course of subsequent chapters. It is useful, therefore, to make them visible at the outset.

Essentially, there are three features of kinship in contemporary society that repay the kind of attention we are giving it here. First, available evidence suggests that kin relationships (outside the immediate household) remain important despite persistent assumptions to the contrary. Second, the changing nature of couple relationships, especially the wider experience of cohabitation, divorce and repartnering, frequently requires a more self-conscious approach to the construction of a kin network. Third, there is growing recognition among social scientists who are not specialists in 'the family' that family relationships lie at the heart of understanding the condition of social life in advanced industrial, or late modern, societies. We shall examine each of these reasons in turn.

First, we observe an almost stubborn persistence of attachment to kin relationships, despite the common wisdom among social scientists that 'the family' means the household and no more, and the apparent acceptance of that view in public discourse. The constraining effects of this definition upon good analysis have been identified by various writers (Finch 1989; Morgan 1996; Jamieson 1998; Smart and Neale 1999). In fact, evidence can be adduced from various sources to demonstrate that most people do place considerable store on family relationships outside the household, including earlier work of our own in which we demonstrated that most people want to believe that they belong to a kin group that 'works' and to feel that they contribute actively to this (Finch and Mason 1993; see also the Family Policy Studies Centre's study of nationally representative British social attitudes data, which supports these arguments: McGlone *et al.* 1998). There is undoubtedly wide variation in who is included in kin groups, what type of interpersonal and practical exchanges are involved and how they change over time. But none of this negates the basic point that there is a widespread conception among the British population that 'my family' means something more than the people with whom I currently share domestic arrangements. It should also be noted that the different cultural traditions represented in this country map onto kin relationships in important ways, even if these are relatively little understood. The broad generalisation that 'the family' has shrunk to its nuclear core never made any sense if it was intended to include British citizens whose cultural roots are in the Indian subcontinent, or Africa, or the Pacific rim (see, for example, Goulbourne 1999).

In summary, these data reveal that there certainly are changes in the ways in which people relate to their kin and, where contact is reducing, it seems to be related to other social changes such as geographical mobility or women's employment. But these changes are within a context of continued high levels of both attachment and contact. Other types of social change are probably more important in understanding the contemporary significance of kinship, which leads to a consideration of our second reason for studying it, namely changing couple relationships.

The commonplace observation that recent decades have seen a major increase in the proportion of people divorcing, remarrying and/or living in non-married cohabitation relationships (with someone of the same or a different sex) has to be balanced against the simple fact that still the majority of marriages do not end in divorce. The rate of divorce rose rapidly in the twenty years following 1971 (when a significant change in the divorce law came into effect) but has levelled off since then. As to cohabitation, most recent figures on heterosexual cohabitation suggest that about one-quarter of unmarried people are living in such a relationship at any given time. However, most of these relationships last for two years or less, and the main reason for their ending is that the partners then marry. Cohabitation was, at least in retrospect, simply a prelude to marriage rather than an alternative (Office for National Statistics 1999: 46–7).

Assumptions about instability in couple relationships therefore do need to be kept in proportion. However, it is certainly true that there is greater diversity of experience of family life among the population, because more people do marry more than once, or live in other types of couple relationship, both heterosexual and non-heterosexual. For a growing proportion of the population, children have a combination of parents and step-parents and potentially, therefore, they have several sets of grandparents, siblings and other kin. Adults also have several sets of potential kin to whom they are linked by in-law (or 'in-law type') relationships. Our understanding of this greater diversity is enhanced by some good new sociological studies (Flowerdew 1999; Smart and Neale 1999; Weeks *et al.* 1999).

The main point that we want to draw from this work at this stage is that, for more people than in the past, explicit and conscious decisions have to be made about who is going to count as 'my family' and for what purpose. It is not that families have been destroyed, rather that they are fashioned and refashioned to suit changing circumstances. This point is developed in an important way by Smart and Neale (1999) in their discussion of 'family fragments', based upon their empirical work on couples with children following a divorce. The emphasis of family law in the 1990s, which prioritises a continuing relationship with both parents, has, they argue, accelerated a tendency for people to construct their own effective 'family' across different households and out of sets of relationships that they have developed at different times and in different contexts. Co-residence can no longer be seen as a universal characteristic even of the nuclear family. The impact of divorce and subsequent unions is to

> disperse the biological family across households and marriages/cohabitations. It may also generate links between grandparents and grandchildren which are no longer anchored in the marriage of the parents but which can survive various transformations in those parents' relationships because they are forged directly with the grandchildren rather than resting on the longevity of the marriage. Moreover in the future these grandparents themselves are likely to be divorced and re-partnered.
>
> (Smart and Neale 1999: 181)

What applies to the particular case of post-divorce grandparenting also applies more generally, as Smart and Neale argue. Drawing upon Morgan's (1996) analysis, they endorse the view that we should no longer be speaking of 'being' part of an institution called 'the family'; rather, we should think about 'doing' family life, actively constructing it out of fragments available to each of us.

These important perspectives on family life, emphasising its active construction even at the level of 'who belongs' to a given family, open up the question of kinship in a new way. When social scientists could make the cosy assertion that nuclear families are coterminous with households and are the only relationships that really count, wider kin relations could be seen as peripheral to contemporary experience. This was always incorrect, as we have argued elsewhere (Finch 1989; Finch and Mason 1993). But the changing nature of the 'nuclear' family, as discussed above, erodes the absolute distinction between family and wider kin and brings kinship back centre stage.

Our third reason for studying kinship is that family life is now much more widely recognised as central to social theory, in particular those social theorists who seek to understand the nature of the individual and the social under conditions of late modernity. The work of Giddens (1991; 1992), Beck (1992), Beck-Gernsheim (Beck and Beck-Gernsheim 1995) and Bauman (1988; 1995) has been particularly influential here.

The starting point for this analysis, which brings families back into mainstream social theory, is the position of individuals under the conditions of late modernity. Giddens speaks of individuals 'forging their self identities' (1991: 1) and 'the reflexive project of the self' (1992: 108). Bauman argues that 'the demise of power-assisted universals and absolutes has made the responsibilities of the actor more profound, indeed more consequential, than ever before' (1995: 6). Beck talks about the 'individualised society', in which each person must consider him or herself 'the centre of action' (1992: 135). The image of individuals constructing their own biographies out of many possible choices is central to this analysis and immediately raises the question of where, if at all, the kinds of commitment that have traditionally been associated with families might fit.

At this point, different answers are possible. Giddens sees intimate relationships as themselves strongly implicated in this project of the reflexive self, arguing that individuals seek to accomplish 'pure relationships', negotiated commitments that last just as long as they are satisfactory and fulfilling. Under conditions of late modernity, the individual has to manage 'the connections between the reflexive project of the self, the pure relationship and the emergence of new ethical programmes for restructuring personal life' (Giddens 1992: 108).

Although he is talking mostly about sexual relationships between couples (whether homo- or heterosexual), he includes kin relationships in this analysis, arguing that these relationships are also bargained and negotiated; commitment in kin relationships is 'as much of an issue as in sexual relationships' (*ibid.*: 96). Beck and Beck-Gernsheim tend to see more of a conflict than Giddens between the position of the individual and family commitments. Indeed, they speak of the family 'breaking apart in the face of the decisions demanded of it' (Beck 1992: 117) and 'a collision between love, the family and personal freedom' (Beck and Beck-Gernsheim 1995: 1). However, this 'collision' occurs mainly with traditional family norms and forms. They see the outcome not as the collapse of families but as radical change in the direction of much greater diversity:

> it is no longer possible to pronounce in some binding way on what family, marriage, parenthood, sexuality or love mean, what they could or should be; rather these vary in substance, exceptions, norms and morality from individual to individual and from relationship to relationship.
>
> (*ibid.*: 5)

From the perspective of our argument here, the most important feature of this work is not the substance of the analysis, which certainly can be questioned (Smart and Neale 1999: 17–19; see also Jamieson 1999 for a critique of Giddens), but the recognition of the significance of family relationships in understanding contemporary social life. Family relationships are seen as important because of the central idea that, in a society where individuals must construct their own lives without many fixed points, close relationships may well be central to the constitution of personal identities.

In summary, therefore, we would argue that there are cogent reasons for trying to understand more about the nature of contemporary kinship. Although we believe that it has always been more important than was often recognised, the changing nature of British society, and the changing ways in which individuals construct their lives, have led to a more widespread recognition of its contemporary significance.

English kinship and inheritance

Although many of the questions about family life raised in this book have resonance in all advanced industrial, or late modern, societies, we have already indicated that we are tying our discussion of inheritance specifically to England because of its distinctive legal framework for transmitting property. The English context is also important when we look at those existing structures and processes that are encompassed by the term 'kinship' and how they have taken on their present form. In essence, English kinship historically has had a distinctive character, and this continues to be profoundly relevant to an understanding of its contemporary forms and meanings. We refer to England specifically because there is insufficient comparative data from within the four countries that comprise the United Kingdom to be certain that the form and meaning of kinship are consistent. Most of the studies, both historical and contemporary, including our own, have been in England; we are therefore being very precise in those points of our discussion where we are focusing upon the English context.

In formal terms, English kinship would be described as bilateral, with descent reckoned through both mother and father, neither of whom is given a privileged position over the other. A series of empirical studies during the second half of the twentieth century have demonstrated that most people operate with a 'concentric circles' model of their own kin, with relationships being most significant between those in the inner circle. We could describe this inner circle as 'intimate' kin, people with whom contact is close and frequent and who are seen to be the most important members of 'my family'; the second circle is made up of intimate kin plus others who are 'effective' kin, people with whom I am in active contact at least at a minimal level, such as sending Christmas cards; the third circle is made up of intimate and effective kin, plus everyone else whose existence I acknowledge but with whom I am not in active contact (Allan 1979; Finch 1989; Finch and Mason 1993; Firth *et al.* 1970; Morgan 1976; Schneider 1968).

From the perspective of the discussion in this book, the most important facet of English kinship as revealed in this literature is not its formal features but the highly flexible way in which people operationalise their own kin relationships within those broad parameters. It is possible to generalise that most people operate a concentric circles model in respect to their own kin. It is not possible to generalise with any degree of certainty about who will be included in which circle. The only feature that is highly predictable is that the inner circle of intimate kin almost always includes 'biological' parents and children, however warm or difficult the actual relationships between the parties. Beyond that, the nature of relationships themselves is important in the 'placing' of an individual relative within one of the circles. It is quite possible, for example, for one brother to be in the inner circle and another not. There is also no necessary mutuality about this; for example, a grandparent may include a grandchild in the inner circle, but the same grandchild may not include the grandparent.

Just as the placing or acknowledgement of kin admits a high degree of variation in the English context, so also is there considerable variation in the nature of these relationships. Maintaining regular contact is an acknowledged feature, but what this means can be highly variable. There are no fixed rules about what one 'must' or 'should' do for even close kin, as our earlier work has shown. Kin relationships are negotiated between the individuals concerned over time, within changing contexts. This does not mean that they are unimportant – far from it. The fact that they are embedded in the personal biographies of the people concerned and the history of the relationship between them gives them a firm, and on many occasions binding, character. But they do not simply follow rules imposed through social custom, convention or law (Finch and Mason 1990a; 1991; 1993).

Where, in the English context, does inheritance fit this picture? We have already noted an important feature of English law, namely the emphasis on testamentary freedom, which means that each person can choose (through the legal mechanism of writing a will) to dispose of property to whoever he or she wishes. When we put this together with the high degree of flexibility in the English kinship system, we can see that inheritance is potentially significant for two reasons. First, it allows individuals to use the act of bequeathing property to define the contours of their own kin relationships, to confirm who 'counts' and what value is placed on each relationship. Second, in the processes of doing this and thinking in advance about doing it, the nature of an individual's kin network is made visible and accessible to the observer, in one of its guises at least. Inheritance is therefore an important way both of studying kinship and, potentially, of constituting kinship. The linked empirical studies that we report in this book have capitalised upon these features.

Having emphasised the potential importance of inheritance to our understanding of kinship, we need to look a bit more closely at the particular perspective on kin relations that it is likely to illuminate. There are two main elements here: first, the material and economic aspects of kinship; second, the more personal and symbolic aspects, linked both to the quality of relationships and to personal identity.

The material and economic importance of inheritance is obvious. It is the means by which wealth (of all types) is passed from one person to another, and over time is the principal means through which the structures of wealth in any society are transmitted, modified and reproduced. There is plenty of evidence that the transmission of wealth across generations has been fundamental to the construction of economic power in the past. As John Scott puts it in his study of the upper classes in Britain, any study of power or privilege brings out

> the continuing importance of the family in the perpetuation of economic privilege. Inheritance remains the major determinant of wealth inequality, as well as the other life chances which depend on this.
>
> (1982: 119)

What was true in the past only for the wealthy minority now applies to the majority of the population, albeit on a more modest scale. At least in principle, the majority of families now have the possibility of wealth building up over several generations as the value of a house is transmitted. Work undertaken by social scientists on current patterns of housing inheritance do indeed show that this is creating patterns in which wealth becomes consolidated within certain families, to the exclusion of others. It is clear from this work that the spread of home ownership is tending to keep wealth within the same sectors of society rather than spreading it more broadly, since, at least at this time, people who are inheriting house property from their parents are already themselves in the owner-occupation section of the housing market. Indeed, it is possible to argue that the ultimate impact of home ownership will be to reinforce the disadvantaged position of that section of the community (about one-fifth at the present time) whose families have not been, and never will be, in a position to own their own homes. Whether this phenomenon is likely to last, or whether it is characteristic of a transitional stage towards a situation where home ownership is spread through the whole population, continues to be a matter of lively debate (see, for example, Forrest and Murie 1995; Hamnett 1991; 1995; Watt 1993; 1996). However, at the moment empirical evidence on home ownership suggests that inheritance reinforces, rather than modifies, the relative economic position of successive generations (Munro 1987).

Looking more generally at how inheritance fits in with the economic role of families, Delphy and Leonard (1992: 151–8) have produced a strong statement about its significance in reproducing social positions, not only between different families but also within each family. Basing their analysis on the situation in both the UK and France, they argue that 'each system of inheritance and transmission is based on advantage/disadvantage and inequality' (*ibid.*: 155). They identify younger sons and all daughters as the people who normally lose out. This analysis presumes a systematic process of disadvantage that reproduces structures of power in the family over time. In their view, it is one of the mechanisms that sustains gender relations on the basis of inequality, as well as shaping life chances according to birth order. There are indeed important questions, which we shall consider in the course of our analysis, about whether children are treated on equal terms with each other. However, whether there are systematic differences according to gender and birth order are questions that we regard as open to empirical investigation, and indeed the answers may well be different in the English and French contexts. Nonetheless, these perspectives are important in highlighting the potential for inheritance to determine the economic context of individuals' lives, as well as to reinforce the economic position of different families.

The second feature of kinship to which inheritance gives access are those less tangible dimensions concerned with the quality of relationships, and the extent to which an individual's own identity is defined and sustained through his or her close relationships. Our own earlier research has shown that kin relationships, and how they are handled, can be critical to personal identity. This earlier work was not about inheritance but about another aspect of kin relationships, namely exchanges of practical, financial and emotional support between family members in a wide range of life circumstances. We found that the dynamic that drives these exchanges in families is bound up in important ways with the identities of the individuals who become involved in them. People's actions towards their kin are part of the process of constructing and maintaining a particular identity – a reliable son, a generous uncle, a caring sister, and so on. Thus, when goods and services are exchanged within families, much more is at stake than material or practical assistance (Finch and Mason 1993). A study of how families handle inheritance, being a process of exchange with high symbolic potential, should give interesting insights into the ways in which identities are constructed and the significance of particular relationships confirmed.

The idea that personal identity is defined increasingly through close relationships is also part of the analysis of late modernity by the writers discussed above. They view this as a feature that is intensifying as individuals increasingly have to take active responsibility for constructing their own lives. Thus Beck and Beck-Gernsheim speak of marriage becoming 'increasingly a matter of identity' (1995: 51) and predict that, in the future 'love ... will turn out to be one of the main sources of satisfaction and meaning in life' (*ibid.*: 169). These perspectives can, as we have argued above, also be considered in respect of other relationships, not just between couples.

Inheritance offers a particular perspective on these qualitative aspects of relationships by drawing in the perspective of time. Family relationships, probably more than any others in which we engage, have time built into their very essence. For example, questions of descent are generally reckoned in terms of kinship, and as Morgan argues, 'family processes and relationships are shaped by and given their dynamism by their linkage to processes of birth, sexuality, death and ageing' (1996: 134). Inheritance of property after someone has died is not simply a practical way of disposing of assets; it can also be a statement about the continuity of relationships. When people reason about how to pass on their property when they die, or about what to do with a legacy received from someone who has died, they are potentially marking boundaries between past, present and future in particular ways that underline this fundamental connection between kinship and time. Possession of objects previously owned by someone who has died potentially gives the living access to a continuing relationship with that person through the phenomenon of memory. Similarly, where a person is contemplating his or her future death, the passing on of objects can potentially become a means of making a statement about the value of particular relationships.

The extent to which objects symbolise relationships over time is something that we explore in later chapters. However, it is a recognised phenomenon in the literature on inheritance – a particularly useful analysis is to be found in the work of the anthropologist Annette Weiner (1992), who writes about the significance of 'inalienable possessions'. Although she draws her data from societies very different from contemporary Britain, principally Papua New Guinea, there are many resonances. In her analysis, inalienable possessions can be anything capable of being transmitted across generations: land rights, material objects, mythic knowledge. These possessions are kept within the family circle, and their loss, if it occurs, diminishes both the individual and the group. The special character of an inalienable possession is that it represents, at one and the same time, both change and continuity, past and future. Their symbolic meaning comes from being given away, passed on to the next generation, yet that meaning is retained only by its association with the person who gave it. Thus, Weiner argues, inalienable possessions are

> the representation of how social identities are reconstituted over time ... the reproduction of kinship is legitimated in each generation by the transmission of inalienable possessions.
> (*ibid.*: 11)

The emphasis here is on the symbolic rather than the material importance of the inalienable possession (some may be materially valuable, others not). Seen in this light, inheritance is fundamentally about the human condition rather than about economic wealth or power. The passing on of inalienable possessions is, in Weiner's analysis,

> grounded in the need to secure permanence in a serial world that is always subject to loss and decay ... [such possessions] bring a vision of permanence into a social world that is always in the process of change. The effort to make memory persist ... is fundamental to nurturing the seeds of change.
> (*ibid.*: 7–8)

Although Weiner's analysis is borne of completely different social conditions from the English context that is our focus, there are reasons to believe that the sense of continuity over time may be if anything an even more important factor here in defining the value of kin relationships. Approaching this issue of continuity from a completely different angle, historian Philippe Aries, in his influential work on the social management of death and dying, confirms the importance of objects and artefacts as providing such continuity. He argues that, in technologically advanced Western societies, death has become a private event where once it was public. From a past in which the death of one individual involved a whole community in public rituals, whether simple or elaborate, marking the loss to that community of the individual who had died, death has now become an event that involves only people intimately connected to the deceased. Sometimes even they are very distant from the event when it takes place in hospital. The increasing popularity of cremation rather than burial further emphasises its private nature, because there is seldom a public memorial. In these circumstances, Aries argues, the 'cult of the tomb' is substituted by the 'cult of memory in the home'. Memory is preserved by keeping certain objects of the deceased in the way in which they were always kept during their lifetime, by buying flowers every year on the deceased's birthday, by keeping a photograph in a prominent place (Aries 1983: 577). This emphasis on memory and continuity stands in sharp contrast to a writer such as Beck, who sees individuals in late modernity focusing on the present and the future – 'the eternal present', as he describes it at one point (1992: 135).

Writing more generally about families and time, Morgan (1996: 142–5) makes some important points about time and memory that have resonance for our own analysis. He argues that family relationships and events mark the passage of time for individuals and give shape to their own biographies in significant ways. Additions and subtractions in family terms are significant markers of the passage of time, and family members engage with each other in 'routine memory work', which marks both the passage of time and the ageing of individuals. It is this shared stock of memories (albeit not always remembered in the same way) that marks out a family or kin group:

Part of what family living means is sharing ... memories of past events and transitions ... Family members, it could be argued, are those who claim certain rights to access the memories of others.

(*ibid.*: 144)

This opportunity for shared memory in families enables people who are not physically present, including those who have died, to continue to be incorporated into family life, Morgan argues. In relation to inheritance, we could extend this argument by postulating that the transmission of objects after the death of an individual, or even in anticipation of that person's death, provides a focus for memory and thereby the greater likelihood that a deceased individual will continue to be part of the family's common stock of memories.

Inheritance therefore gives us a particular purchase on understanding contemporary kinship that illuminates it from particular angles. The features thus illuminated have particular resonance because kin relationships potentially offer a network in which an individual's identity can be constituted, and which can be durable over time. The English context provides a particularly rich vehicle for this, we have argued, because of the flexibility afforded both by kinship 'structures' and by the legal context.

Kinship, individualism and relationism

There are, as we have shown, a range of important questions about contemporary kinship that repay empirical exploration. In developing these within the particular perspective of inheritance, we believe that a valuable starting point is the concept of individualism.

We have already noted that English kinship is characterised by a high degree of flexibility and choice. Some recent writings on kinship have deployed the idea of individualism to conceptualise this. Whether or not the actual word is used, we believe that much of the most significant scholarly work on English kinship has some kind of concept of individualism at its heart. Furthermore, a concept of individualism has been more or less central to the recent influential writing on late modernity on which we have drawn (especially Beck 1992; but also Giddens 1991; Bauman 1988; 1995). We believe therefore that a discussion of what is meant by individualism in these contexts is an important and potentially useful starting point for our study of kinship and inheritance. We begin by considering the ways in which the concept of 'individualism' has been used in social science to apply – explicitly or potentially – to kinship.

In contemporary analyses of English kinship, the most important source of discussions of individualism is in the writing of Marilyn Strathern and her colleagues (Strathern 1992; Edwards *et al.* 1993), growing out of their empirical work on the technologies of assisted conception and what these mean for the ways in which people understand kinship and family. The background to their analyses is classic social anthropology, in which understanding kinship in any society focuses upon mapping the relationship between positions in a genealogical table. Against this background, Strathern argues that English kinship is distinctively individualistic, by which she means that, among other things, individuals do not relate to each other simply by virtue of their genealogical position. This means that a child, for example, is not regarded simply as 'a son' or 'a daughter' but as a unique individual. Relationships between kin operate not purely on the basis of 'positions' but between 'persons'. The implication is that knowing someone to be my brother or my aunt reveals little about the type of relationship that I have with that person; rather, it depends *which* brother or aunt. Crucially, however, Strathern's vision is not of a society of atomised individuals, because the very idea of individualism comes *from* relationships and their social meaning and, in that sense, is produced *by* kinship:

> the particular social relationship of parent and child generates the image of the child not just as a son or daughter but as a unique individual. Indeed, we might consider *the individuality of persons as the first fact of English kinship*.
> (Strathern 1992: 14; italics in original)

In a strong sense, then, Strathern's 'first fact of English kinship' constitutes a rejection of the idea of formal and predictable kinship structures based on genealogical position, but *not* of the salience of kin relations. This formulation is extremely valuable in analytical terms. In the context of our own work, we would want to suspend judgement for the moment about whether there is an absolute distinction between 'persons' and 'positions', or whether there are circumstances in which the two intersect. Nonetheless, a strong emphasis on 'persons' and a corresponding de-emphasis on 'positions' would seem to be the core feature of English kinship, which in many ways sets it apart from other European kinship systems.

Strathern draws on the influential work of the historian Alan Macfarlane in her analysis, and we too have found a stimulus in some of his ideas on the origins of English individualism. Macfarlane describes English kinship as 'ego-centred', in the sense that each individual is at the centre of his or her own kin universe and kinship is reckoned outwards from oneself. He contrasts this with 'ancestor-centred' kinship, in which kinship is reckoned by tracing a lineage back to an ancestor. Individualism, in this sense, means *the very structure of the kin group*, the idea of concentric circles with one person in the middle. It underlines the fundamental point that no two individuals have precisely the same kin network; each individual constructs his or her own. Unlike many other kinship systems, there is no sense of a family that pre-exists and that an individual can 'join'. In the English context, it has long been the case that an individual expects to create a family, not to join one (Macfarlane 1978).

Macfarlane's work is one of the very few examples in the literature on individualism that is explicitly concerned with property ownership and its historical relationship to families. Indeed, his whole project is a debate with the orthodox analysis (attributed to Marx and Weber) of property ownership over time, in which it was presumed that England in the past was essentially a peasant society with associated structures of land ownership and property rights. If this were true, Macfarlane argues, then property ownership should have had two characteristics: property rights reside essentially with the family, not with individuals; property remains with the 'community of males', with women having no opportunities to own and dispose of property. Macfarlane argues that the historical evidence does not support this view of property ownership in England (*ibid.*: 131–5).

This brings an additional insight to our analysis of English kinship, namely that arrangements for property ownership and transmission are themselves pointers to individualism. Extrapolating from Macfarlane's historical analysis, we can argue that an individualistic kinship structure can be characterised by certain types of property ownership. In particular, property is held by the individual, who has full rights to use and dispose of it. The contrast here is with a situation where individuals hold property in trust for, or on behalf of, the family as a whole. This latter view is neatly encapsulated in the concept of 'patrimony', which is a concept widely understood in some other European countries. For example, writing against the background of the French experience, Delphy and Leonard describe it as

> Patrimony is 'the property of the family' but it is held at any one time by individuals and is passed on by them ... to other individuals ... Holding the property gives the person concerned power and advantages.
>
> (1992: 157)

Historically, this form of what we might call 'transgenerational ownership' has never been close to the English experience, according to Macfarlane. In relation to our own study, the questions of whether there is a strong or weak concept of 'family property', and whether or not distinctions are made between women and men as holders and transmitters of property, should therefore provide a useful indicator of the nature and degree of individualism in English.

These ideas about individualism and the structure of English kinship are, therefore, potentially very useful for our analysis of kinship and inheritance. But there are other uses of the concept of individualism from which we would wish to maintain a greater distance, and yet which have a relevance for our discussion here. These are found in the concept of individualism used in more recent sociological writing, which focuses on the position of the individual in late modernity, although we should point out that family relationships tend to be one part of the analysis here rather than its central focus. Echoing Macfarlane's work, Beck writes that individuals now have to learn to construct their own lives and biographies within a social world where each must see him or herself as the centre:

> In an individualised society the individual must learn ... to conceive of himself or herself as the centre of action, as the planning office with respect to his/her own biography, abilities, orientations and relationships.
>
> (1992: 135)

In Beck's analysis, the driving force for this ego-centred world is the requirements of the labour market and of being a consumer. A different slant is put by Bauman, who tends to see it as in part a cultural phenomenon in which individuals are expected to build up their identities in a positive and conscious fashion. He describes it as 'an impulse to look on one's own "self" as an object of tender care and cultivation' (Bauman 1988: 36)

The common ground in all these writings is an agreement that the current state of the human condition in advanced industrial, or late modern, societies is that 'the reflexive project of the self', as Giddens calls it, becomes the central aim of life. The implication of this analysis is that individualism means not just that each person is the centre of his or her own world but also that this is how it *should be*. There is a legitimacy about being ego-centred that is a requirement of contemporary living. Cultivating one's own identity is central to acting as a social being but may, as we have noted above, require close personal relationships to be developed and sustained.

There is a clear sense in this writing that something has changed in the last couple of decades: a removal of prescribed social formulae for living; a loss of security, which once came through accepted social norms; and a new type of relationship of the individual to society as a whole. Essentially, what is being argued here is not that individualism is completely new but that it has undergone a kind of intensification, becoming more required than optional, and being relevant to much wider sections of the population than in the past. The family and intimacy are seen as undergoing transformation in this context: Giddens speaks of kinship relations that 'used to be taken for granted as the basis of trust' (1992: 96). Beck and Beck-Gernsheim write that 'time honoured norms are fading' in families (1995: 7) and that the 'traditional unity' of the family is 'breaking apart' (*ibid.*: 117).

This formulation of individualism has two main limitations for our purposes. The first concerns the suggestion that individualism (in kinship and elsewhere) is a recent development. However, Macfarlane and others have argued that an historical analysis shows that the individualistic character of English kinship has long existed. It is by no means a recent phenomenon. There are, not surprisingly, different accounts of how and when English kinship took on its distinctively individualistic character. Stone identifies individualistic features in the type of family being established in the sixteenth and seventeenth centuries (1977). Macfarlane dates its origins at least to the thirteenth century, but the main point of his argument is that in England the primary social world has long revolved around the individual, rather than providing fixed groups into which individuals must fit.

But as well as disputing the accuracy of the historical bases of some of the more recent sociological claims about individualism in relation to kinship systems, there are some problems with their contemporary application. The main difficulty here, as Mason has argued elsewhere, is with the implication that the individual is a singular 'prime mover' in these accounts (Mason 2000: 5). This 'individual' is very different to the 'individuality' at the centre of Strathern's view of English kinship, which was constructed against a backdrop of conventional anthropological understandings of kinship as a system of genealogical positions. Strathern's individuality is the product of relationships and of kinship, and it allows for the formulation of kinship as based more on persons than genealogical positions. In contemporary sociological writing, however, the individual is seen as the prime mover in the project of the self. Relationships are important, but only as adjuncts to this overall project. However, as Mason points out, this version of the individual as prime mover is at odds with contemporary empirical evidence (including our own earlier work: Finch and Mason 1993), as well as alternative theorisations of the social relations and moralities of late modernity (Sevenhuijsen 1998), which point to more connected, more relational, forms of social existence. She suggests not only that kin relationships and commitments are much more central and enduring in people's lives than is implied by these writers but also that the very notion of the 'project of the self' may have significantly less contemporary empirical and theoretical resonance than an idea of relational projects, and relational biographies, based on a *reflexive relationism* rather than a reflexive individualism. If that is the case, then it may be more useful to try to understand how relationism, rather than individualism, operates in the context of kinship and inheritance.

The 'Inheritance Study' and the shape of the book

Having set out the particular orientations of our study and some of the influences on our thinking, we now move to a series of chapters in which we explore the contemporary significance of kinship, as looked at from the perspective of how inheritance is handled in England. To do this, we use data from our three linked empirical studies. Further details of the study and the methodology are contained in Appendix A. The three elements are:

1 The analysis of a randomly selected sample of 800 probated wills from people who died in the years 1959, 1969, 1979 and 1989. Our reason for selecting these four sample years was to enable us to see whether there have been any changes in the pattern of bequeathing over that period when the rate of home ownership has been rising.
2 A set of eighty-eight in-depth interviews with ninety-eight people, male and female, about how inheritance issues are handled in practice within families. The interviewees were selected on the basis that they came from 'ordinary' as opposed to wealthy families, but otherwise they covered a reasonable spread of socio-economic circumstances, including housing tenure. Fifteen were of Asian origin, and two were white British married to someone of Asian origin. The rest were white British. Their ages ranged from 18 to 89. They all lived in England, most but not all in the north of England, at the time of the interview, but their places of origin were quite widely varied and included some from the Indian subcontinent. Thirty-two interviewees were in the study as individuals, and the remaining sixty-six had one or more members of their own family who also was. Our largest family group in the study included eight interviewees.
3 A set of thirty semi-structured interviews with solicitors and other professionals who dealt with making wills, inheritance and probate. We selected professionals from a range of types and sizes of legal or financial institution, based in the north of England and the Midlands. Again, we interviewed both men and women.

We use these data to pursue a number of questions about kinship and inheritance, and our discussions both develop themes raised in this chapter and bring other issues and perspectives into the frame. Chapter 2 demonstrates some of the complexities of inheritance through a detailed analysis of the 'case study' of divorce, separation, repartnering and step-families, and it opens up further questions about kinship which are addressed in the rest of the book. Chapter 3 gives an overview of how property is transmitted and divided in families through the process of inheritance. Chapter 4 shifts the focus onto receiving an inheritance and examines what our data on inheriting money tell us about moralities of kinship. Chapter 5 explores questions of ownership in the inheritance process, and what these reveal about kinship, by examining how people handle and reason about potential conflicts between financing old age and preserving assets to pass on to family. Chapter 6 focuses on symbolic dimensions of inheritance and examines the centrality of the 'keepsake' in people's understandings of what inheritance and kinship are about. Finally, Chapter 7 pulls together the key themes of the book in a discussion of what inheritance tells us about how we should understand contemporary English kinship.

Chapter 2

Questions of complexity
A case study

Introduction

We begin our empirical exploration of kinship and inheritance by way of a case study of a very specific issue, namely inheritance in families where there has been a history that includes divorce, cohabitation following divorce, remarriage, step-relationships or a combination of these experiences. We are calling these 'complex families', since other terms like 'reconstituted families' fail to capture the diversity and fluidity of family practices in these circumstances (Smart and Neale 1999). We do not mean to suggest that these situations represent the norm for English families, although they are increasingly common, as we noted in Chapter 1. However, we believe that the management of inheritance in these families can illuminate priorities and processes that are more generally applicable.

In these families, inheritance questions arise in a particularly complex form, especially given the freedom that English law allows to include and exclude. It is thus possible, in a way that it is not under some other jurisdictions, to use inheritance to define the boundaries of kinship to allow for reconstitution of the network through a series of marriages and marriage-like relationships. Do people ever bequeath to former spouses? Conversely, do they take steps specifically to exclude former spouses? Is a second spouse treated, for purposes of inheritance, as if she or he was the first spouse? How are step-children treated? Are they included on the same terms as children with a genetic link or excluded altogether, or included on different terms?

These are points at which individualism and relationism should be clearly visible if they are important in English kinship. Families with experience of divorce, separation, repartnering and step-relationships should help us to test some of the key ideas that we introduced in Chapter 1: are persons more important than positions? In what sense does 'the family' have a common stake in property? To what extent is inheritance part of a 'project of the self' or conversely a 'reflexive relationism'? We are therefore using these complex families as a case study to open up a perspective upon the topic of inheritance and kinship more generally. In the course of this chapter, we shall identify themes that will be explored more extensively in subsequent chapters.

Writing a will in a complex family

The significance of inheritance when people have been divorced and/or remarried is prominent in our interviews with solicitors. More than half identified divorce and remarriage as circumstances where they would always advise clients to make a will; some make it a rule always to raise the question as part of divorce proceedings. From a legal perspective, there are various pitfalls that can be anticipated, and, solicitors argue, a will should be written to ensure that the outcome in practice is in accordance with the client's wishes. The examples mentioned to us included the possibility that a divorced spouse may make a claim on the estate under certain conditions; that property might pass to the children of the second marriage, excluding any from the first marriage of either partner; that a second spouse who is the survivor of the marriage might dispose of property that had previously been jointly owned, thus excluding children from the deceased spouse's previous marriage. These are possibilities that also concern the people whom we interviewed in relation to their own families, as we shall show later in this chapter.

One might expect therefore that wills would tell us a good deal about how divorce, remarriage and the creation of step-families are treated for inheritance purposes. In fact, this is not the case. Our data from the sample of 800 wills yields very little about bequeathing within these kinds of families, partly because a will never tells us who is excluded. The following extract, in which the will states explicitly that the testator's estranged wife and son should receive nothing, is a very unusual – albeit intriguing – case:

Nothing must go to my wife Mrs. Millbank whom I have not seen for many years as I have been legally separated *by Court* and don't know her whereabouts. Also nothing must be given to my son who I have never seen since he was a baby.

(italics in original)

Wills are normally silent on such matters. We do find that there are a few cases where step-children are named as beneficiaries, however, so we know that they are included by at least some testators. A total of sixteen wills (2 per cent of the sample) name a step-relative either as a beneficiary or as a substitute in the event of the first-choice beneficiary dying before the testator. Thirteen step-children appear as first-choice beneficiaries, five of whom receive cash gifts, but the remaining eight receive a share of the total or residuary estate and – in one case – the testator's home. These 'major' gifts are normally associated with children rather than more distant kin, so in this small number of wills where step-children are mentioned, the majority are treated in the same way as children. When they appear in wills as substitutes, they are mostly designated to take the share of a major gift that would have gone to their own parent, who in most cases would be the second spouse of the testator. Again, this is a typical formula for children. So, where step-children do appear in wills, their treatment is analogous to children. Of course, we have no way of knowing how many of our testators had step-children who got nothing. It may well be that, in the future, many more wills will explicitly include bequests to step-children as the increased number of people divorced and remarried in the last quarter of the twentieth century reaches old age.

Wills therefore give us relatively few clues about inheritance within complex families. However, our data from interviews do tell us a considerable amount about how people are beginning to incorporate second marriages and step-relationships into their thinking about inheritance. In selecting our study population, we deliberately tried to include a significant number of people who had direct experience in their own families of divorce or remarriage or step-relationships. In total, there are thirty-two people who have such experience. In addition, another fourteen have experienced one or more of these within their wider kin group.

As we have already noted, logically the complexities of arranging inheritance where divorce, separation, repartnering and step-relationships are part of the scene should lead people to write a will. However, by no means all of our interviewees with experience of divorce and remarriage had done so. Among those respondents who have had direct experience of divorce, remarriage or cohabitation, nine had written a will but seven had not. If we exclude interviewees aged over 60, where there is much greater likelihood that a person will have written a will (see Chapter 3), those who have not written a will (seven) marginally outnumber those who have (five). If we take all who have experience of complex families in some form or other, it is clear that this is not leading them towards making a will. Again excluding people over 60, six interviewees had written a will, but twenty-one had not.

Thus a close acquaintance with the complexities of life in divorce, separation, repartnering or step-relationships does not trigger a desire to sort out one's own inheritance affairs, even where interviewees were aware that they were storing up potential problems. For example, Elizabeth Osborne, who told us that she had not written a will, responded as follows to a question about doing so:

INTERVIEWER: Have you given any thought, or have you discussed with your husband, about how you want to write a will?
ELIZABETH: No, not really. I suppose one of these days we'll have to get round to it.
INTERVIEWER: Do you know what would happen if you died without a will?
ELIZABETH: Oh there would probably be one hell of a problem I should think, sorting everything out.
(Elizabeth Osborne, 40s, second marriage, second-generation home owner)

Elizabeth is almost certainly correct that there would be 'one hell of a problem' if she and her husband were to die intestate. Both have been married before. She has two young sons from her first marriage (who now live with herself and her second husband). He also has two children from his previous marriage, both of whom are adult and living independently. Relationships with his two older children are not as warm as Elizabeth would like, although there never appears to have been any specific argument or break with them.

Inheritance issues in this family are complicated in a variety of ways. There are issues raised by having two cohorts of children, one grown-up and the other not, because children who are dependent upon their parents at the time of death would have a strong claim on the estate. If, therefore, Elizabeth and her husband wish the two older children to inherit anything, they need specifically to provide for that. However, it would seem that she and her husband are likely to take different views on this topic. Although she does not have a close relationship with the two older children, Elizabeth says that she would nonetheless want to treat them on equal terms with the younger ones ('I should hope it would go equally between the four of them'). However, she thinks that her husband would take a different view. She believes that he would wish to provide for the two younger children in preference to his own if they were to die while the children were still living in their home. Unlike her relationship with his children, he has a close relationship with hers ('They are very good. They call him Dad. They consider him as their Dad'). We therefore have a situation that is not only complex in legal terms but also where the two partners' wishes appear to differ. Rationally, Elizabeth and her husband should find themselves a solicitor as quickly as possible. But they have not, possibly precisely because of the difficult issues surrounding their family situation, which would have to be faced if their wishes are to be expressed in legal form.

Although many people, like Elizabeth Osborne, have not yet fully resolved the inheritance implications of being in a complex family, some have thought it through with great care. Most of our interviewees have some outline ideas about what they want to happen, and how that links to the current shape of their family, but they are still in the process of working it all out. This is valuable for our analysis, because it makes visible the underlying principles or guidelines that people are trying to deploy to resolve the particular complexities of their own situations. It is data of this type, rather than what people put into their wills, that we shall use to structure the discussion in the rest of this chapter.

'Passing out of the family': a narrative

In analysing our data about divorce and remarriage, and their impact on inheritance, it becomes clear that the dominant theme – whether from people who have had direct experience or from others – is to avoid money 'passing out of the family', as a consequence of remarriage in particular. This enables us to explore how far there is a 'family stake' in property and how boundaries are drawn around 'the family' for this purpose.

We develop our central theme by setting out in *narrative* form the scenario that our interviewees worry about. We use the concept of narrative here and throughout the book as a methodological and analytical device to communicate what we think are shared cultural meanings and values about kinship and inheritance, which we have drawn out of our interview data. Our narratives are composite ones; they are built up from stories that people told about their own experiences, about the experiences of others known to them, and from comments that people made about the kinds of situation that they hoped to avoid in future. They are not intended to represent a composite story of what happens, or of what people do, in individual cases. Indeed, this particular composite narrative about money 'passing out of the family', and the variations that follow, is constructed out of people's hopes and fears as much as – usually more than – direct experience. As we shall show, people's own practices are constructed in part through engagement with the narrative, and often in opposition to it. They are in no sense a direct reflection of it. However, the ways in which people express their concerns – which we have formulated into a composite narrative – give a clear insight into how they think of 'the family' for inheritance purposes, and of what they think is morally appropriate and inappropriate, whether or not the precise circumstances described have ever occurred in their lives.

We have written this particular narrative so that it is a woman's estate that is in question; it could equally be a man's. The basic narrative runs like this:

Basic narrative
1   Jane marries John (Jane/John marriage).
2   They have children (Jane/John children).
3   The Jane/John marriage ends in divorce.
4   Jane marries Robert (Jane/Robert marriage).
5   Jane dies.
6   As the surviving spouse, Robert inherits everything from Jane.
7   Robert dies.

8   Property is distributed in a way that excludes Jane/John children.
Thus Jane's money has 'passed out of the family'.

What does this narrative tell us about the meanings of family and inheritance in complex family contexts? The first and most obvious is that spouses and children form the core of an individual's family for inheritance purposes, but of the two the spouse is accorded primacy. The pivotal point in the narrative is where Jane dies and the surviving spouse takes everything. This is where the trouble begins, because the principle of the surviving spouse taking everything – relatively unproblematic where the two partners have only ever been married to each other – clashes with the other principle operating in this narrative, namely that priority is given to direct descendants.

When people speak about money 'passing out of the family', the family means Jane's own children. If Robert, as the second spouse, has an estate to bequeath and if any of his remaining assets could be 'traced' to Jane's estate, then there is a strong feeling that any Jane/John children should get some benefit. If they do not, Jane's money has passed out of the family.

However, it is by no means as simple as equating 'family' with 'children'. We can take the analysis a little further by probing the relative claims of Jane/John children, of Robert (the second spouse) of Robert's kin, and of any children who may have been born to the second marriage. We can do this by examining variations on the basic narrative, also found within our data set:

Variation 1
(begins as in basic narrative)
1   Jane marries John (Jane/John marriage).
2   They have children (Jane/John children).
3   The Jane/John marriage ends in divorce.
4   Jane marries Robert (Jane/Robert marriage).
(changes here)
5   Jane anticipates that she might die first, so she writes a will that ensures that both Robert and the Jane/John children benefit.
Thus Jane's money has not 'passed out of the family', because the Jane/John children eventually inherit some of it.

In Variation 1, the children of the first marriage (Jane/John children) do not inherit everything, and they probably receive less than they would have done if their parent had not married a second time, since Jane has taken action to protect the interests of her second spouse as well as her children. However, this is regarded as reasonable by our interviewees. It is quite acceptable that Robert, the second husband, should benefit. The key point is that Jane has taken steps to ensure that her own children receive something from their mother's estate rather than give Robert complete control, thereby running the risk that they would get nothing. What they actually receive has been her choice, their mother having exercised testamentary freedom, which is both her right and – it would seem from this version of the narrative – her responsibility.

The other two variations pose scenarios that are considerably more complex. Variation 2 introduces two more sets of children into the picture, creating complex step-parent and half-sibling relationships:

Variation 2
(begins as in basic narrative)
1 Jane marries John (Jane/John marriage).
2 They have children (Jane/John children).
3 The Jane/John marriage ends in divorce.
4 Jane marries Robert (Jane/Robert marriage).
(changes here)
5 Robert already has children from another marriage (Robert/Susan children).
6 Jane and Robert have children.
7 Jane dies.
8 As the surviving spouse, Robert inherits everything from Jane.
9 Robert dies.
10 Property is distributed between Robert's children (Robert/Susan and Jane/Robert children).
Thus Jane's money has 'passed out of the family', despite the fact that some of her children (Jane/Robert children) do inherit, because others (Jane/John children) do not.

In Variation 2, step-children are included as part of 'the family' within which money is kept. Provided that direct descendants receive something, it is accepted that proportions of Jane's estate can legitimately go to Robert/Susan children, with whom Jane has no genetic relationship. It would be best if *all* Jane's own children receive something. However, the main point is that people see it as legitimate to acknowledge step-children as part of 'the family' for inheritance purposes, depending on the circumstances. As we illustrate below, the critical factor seems to be whether the step-parent has formed a personal and warm relationship with a step-child, either in the latter's childhood or in adult life. In these circumstances, it appears to be seen as natural for that relationship to be acknowledged through inheritance. The essential point is that it is the type of relationship formed with the step-child, not the formal link through remarriage, that counts.

The significance of this point about the character of personal relationships is further reinforced in Variation 3, which represents the ultimate 'horror story' about money passing out of the family:

Variation 3
(begins as in basic narrative)
1   Jane marries John (Jane/John marriage).
2   They have children (Jane/John children).
3   The Jane/John marriage ends in divorce.
4   Jane marries Robert (Jane/Robert marriage).
5   Jane dies.
6   As the surviving spouse, Robert inherits everything from Jane.
(changes here)
7   Robert marries Clare.
8   Robert dies.
9   As the surviving spouse, Clare inherits everything from Robert (which includes what remains of Jane's estate).
10 Clare dies.
11 Clare's property is distributed within her family.
Thus not only has Jane's money 'passed out of the family' but it has ended up with people who had no personal knowledge of Jane.

The horror element is that the people who ultimately benefit *never knew* Jane, from whom the money originates. There is no claim based on a genetic link or any personal relationship between testator and beneficiary. Although our interviewees do not necessarily hold Clare's family culpable, morally they regard it as an aberration that they should inherit any of Jane's estate, especially if this means that Jane's children get nothing. In a situation where there are children who could have inherited, it is the lack of personal relationship that makes this into a horror story.

This composite narrative, with its variations, reveals a complex scenario in which a number of considerations come into play in the shaping of inheritance within complex families:

- the commitments associated with marriage;
- the importance of the genetic link with direct descendants;
- the legitimacy accorded to step-relationships based upon direct personal interaction;
- a corresponding lack of legitimacy for relationships that happen to have a genetic link but no direct personal relationship; and
- the significance of testamentary freedom, which is both a right and a responsibility.

In individual cases in our data we can see people juggling with all of these issues as they work through, in their own particular circumstances, both issues related to inheritance and the definition and redefinition of kinship that this exercise entails.

Inheritance and kinship in complex families

What does this narrative tell us about inheritance in families with experience of divorce, separation, repartnering or step-relationships, and through this the nature of kinship? In exploring these issues, we shall use data from our interviews that allow us *inter alia* to illustrate how our narrative is derived from the experiences of our interviewees. However, it is important to remember that this narrative is not simply a convenient way of summarising our interviewees' experiences of handling inheritance within complex families. It is a narrative that people recognise, and with which they identify, irrespective of whether their own circumstances parallel any of the variants. It is a way in which shared cultural meanings and values can be expressed. The narrative forms a kind of backdrop against which individuals work out their own lives.

Spouses

When it comes to inheritance, the main problem for complex families is that there has been a second wife or husband (sometimes more than two). At first sight, this looks like a banal observation. In fact it is rather an important conclusion that emerges from our data. To put it another way: *the difficulties are created by remarriage, not by divorce.* In our narrative, the trouble starts *not* when Jane and John's marriage ends but when Jane remarries.

Divorce itself does not disturb the *balance* between the claims of a spouse and the claims of children. Either the spouse retains some claims on joint property (normally settled as part of divorce proceedings) or the divorce simply reinforces the claims of the children by removing the divorced spouse from the scene completely. In this case, it would make no difference if the Jane/John marriage had been ended by divorce or by the death of John. The situation is exactly the same. Tensions between the claims of the (second) spouse and Jane's children only arise once Jane remarries, and the tensions would be precisely the same whether that marriage took place after a divorce or the death of the first partner.

An example of this conflict developing in practice comes from Angela Sale, one of our interviewees who had been divorced and was cohabiting with a second partner. In this extract, she is talking about her mother, who had been divorced, remarried and was now separated from her second husband. In the course of the second marriage, her step-father acquired access to her mother's assets, although, as Angela puts it, this was 'covered up' by a pretence that he had actually sunk in money of his own:

INTERVIEWER: Did (your mother) write that will when she divorced the first time?
ANGELA: I think it was when she remarried that the will was written.
INTERVIEWER: And was that when she put most of the money into the second house?
ANGELA: Yes.
INTERVIEWER: So how did you feel about that going to him, as it were?
ANGELA: Well there was a lot of, like, cover-up that he'd put money in there – and he hadn't. We knew he hadn't. But that

was up to her really. I wasn't very pleased, but that was her mistake and she'll pay for it now.

(Angela Sale, late 20s, divorced and cohabiting, second-generation home owner)

In Angela's account, the spouse–children conflict is focused explicitly on remarriage, since this was the point at which her mother wrote a will favouring her new husband and including a house that she had just purchased. Her mother was obviously aware of the tensions that this created with her own children since, according to Angela, she tried to pretend that her new husband had contributed to the purchase. Had that been the case, Angela would have presumed no claim over what her step-father had brought into the marriage. As it was, she felt that she had lost out ('I wasn't very pleased') on assets that might eventually have been hers. She blames her mother for this and appears to believe that some rough justice has been done ('She'll pay for it now') through the subsequent ending of that marriage, in which, presumably, her mother herself lost rights over what she brought to the marriage.

The tensions to which we refer have a distinctive flavour under English legal regimes because of the combination of testamentary freedom with an increasing tendency to emphasise the rights of a spouse (Finch *et al.* 1996). It is this combination that contains the seeds of tension between children and second spouse. Other legal systems, which unambiguously privilege children in inheritance law, cannot create the same kind of difficulty.

English law allows the opportunity to accord the spouse a privileged position. In practice, the claims of a spouse are frequently treated as having priority over the claims of children. Our data show this clearly, and we shall explore this issue more generally in Chapter 3. Typically, a spouse will receive the whole estate, or the estate minus some very small gifts that have been left to others. This applies to a surviving second spouse as much as to a first; for the most part no distinction is made. This is possible because the claims of the first spouse would normally be settled at the time of the divorce.

Although there may be no continuing claim from the first *spouse*, there is a sense in which the first *marriage* still exercises claims, according to the thinking that our interviewees display. People reason that in the course of the first marriage resources were accumulated to which children of that marriage have some claim. Our interviewees are particularly troubled by the prospects of these 'first marriage' resources passing under the control of the second spouse and thence 'out of the family'. This is the whole point of our composite narrative, in all its versions. It is the assets that Jane brought from her marriage to John that are at issue, not any additional resources that she acquired during her marriage to Robert.

Thus there is an interesting sense in which first and second marriages are not quite equivalent for inheritance purposes. In first marriages, there is an assumption that, being at an early stage of their lives, neither partner brings much in the way of assets and that the couple then subsequently build their asset base together, as a joint enterprise. However, it is different in second marriages. One or both may have built up quite significant resources through a previous marriage simply because they are older and more established. The partners therefore do not necessarily enter the marriage on equal terms, especially if there is an age difference. As a consequence, the claims of a second spouse on the resources that have been built up in the previous marriage are ambiguous. Furthermore, depending somewhat on the ages of the parties at the time of the second marriage, the arrangements may not be expected to last very long and will be at a time of life when assets are as likely to be drawn upon as to be built up. So there is a sense in which people want to treat second marriages as an arrangement where the spouses' resources are kept separate, conceptually if not on a day-to-day basis.

Evidence for this analysis comes through in several ways. Jennifer Murray articulates it when she says that she talks about the special circumstances of people marrying 'later in life':

INTERVIEWER: You were saying that ... if you wrote a will you might want to include something about remarriage.
JENNIFER: Oh yes! I did wonder about that, you know. More people [now] marry later on, if their partner has died, where at one time they would stay on their own. There seem to be more incidents of people marrying late in life, even though they know it's just going to be for a few years probably. I feel that I don't want my contribution, economic contribution in this house going towards their family.

(Jennifer Murray, 40s, second marriage, home owner)

Jennifer, currently in her second marriage, anticipates that she might die before her husband and that he might remarry quite 'late in life'. In those circumstances, which she regards as more common now than in the past, she would want her own assets ring-fenced and not to pass to her husband's next spouse on his death. The placing of 'late' marriages in the life course ('there seem to be more incidents of people marrying later in life') and the likely length of the relationship before death intervenes ('even though they know it's just going to be for a few years') combine to make her view these as a *special category* of marriages for inheritance purposes. Angela Sale makes a similar point when she talks about the arrangements for her own current cohabitee, who has moved into the home that she owns and also shares with the children of her first marriage:

> I'd like them all to live here together, Mark and the children. And then when anything happened to him or if he remarried, the house could be sold and divided between the children.
> (Angela Sale, late 20s, divorced and cohabiting, home owner)

Angela – possibly drawing lessons from her mother's experience quoted above – makes it clear that, although she would want to provide for Mark during his lifetime, she regards him as having no ultimate claim on her estate. She has built up the assets, and they should be for her children, commenting that this is more important to her than 'thinking about a fella's feelings'. Like Jennifer Murray, she instinctively wants to move to Variation 2 of our narrative, where action is taken to ensure that money does not pass out of the family and that her children will benefit. However, neither has actually made a will yet.

Using a similar logic, some interviewees go to considerable lengths to work through how assets can be kept separate, in recognition that second marriages (or marriage-like relationships) are not the same as first ones. One way of doing this is to explicitly 'draw a line' under the assets of the first marriage and to treat the children of that marriage as having an exclusive claim to any property acquired during it. An example of this comes from our interview with Sandra Thompson and Paul Watson, who are currently cohabiting. Both have children from previous marriages, Sandra having been divorced and Paul having been widowed. As we observed above, the issues that they face are entirely equivalent.

Questions of complexity

Paul and Sandra explained that they have a rather elaborate plan for distributing the assets of their previous marriages to their respective children, although they have not yet put this arrangement into effect by writing wills. This includes making an assessment of how much capital each brought into the relationship and invested in the purchase of their present house. In their view, that capital sum needs to be preserved for the children through whatever series of financial transactions may occur in the future. But the line is drawn once the previous marriages ended, and the children do not have any equivalent claims over assets that he and Sandra may generate together.

PAUL: Even the house we live in, if we want to leave it, the money that is left from the transaction will be split up 40/60 out of 50/50. The cash would be in the bank ... [and if one of us died] the cash that belonged to the partner that was dead would have to be there, in a trust, except that it could be used if it was really needed.

SANDRA: It's just so that both our children will benefit from what their own particular families have worked so hard to achieve ...

PAUL: And whatever we made from now on wouldn't count. It's just the basic, what we go in at, [in the right] percentage.
(Sandra Thompson and Paul Watson, both 50s, both divorced and cohabiting, home owners)

From examples like this we can see that, although people seek to apply the principle that a spouse's claims override others to second marriages, there is also a recognition that circumstances do change as people move through different marriages. The assets that people bring into each new relationship are bound to be different from those that they brought into the previous one. Thus we see, from the case of complex families, that not only relationships change over time. Property also changes. The property that any individual possesses can both accumulate and diminish as he or she passes through their life course. This has to be taken into account when people are working out the different claims that others have upon them – and they upon others – at different periods of their lives.

Children

Despite the important messages about spouses, the focus of our composite narrative is clearly upon children. There is a presumption throughout all versions of the narrative in favour of the children's claims on their mother's estate. This is fundamental to the point of the story. Thus, despite the lack of legal claims accorded to children under British law, the whole point of this story is that it is unfair if children do not inherit. In this sense, the descent line does have a special status.

The messages about children's claims are, however, rather subtle. What we are seeing is not really a straightforward statement about the rights of children to have property passed on to them by their parents. The message is actually more complex and more conditional. We shall explore this by looking at two aspects of the story, and one other that is not covered explicitly:

- whether children have the right to expect that property will be preserved for them;
- treatment of children and step-children;
- the type of property that should be passed on.

The right to expect

In our composite narrative, the emotion is generated by the prospect of money 'passing out of the family'. This is not the same thing as saying that parents should make sure that there are assets to be passed on to children when they die. If money is there, it should be kept in the family; but it may already have been spent. This seems to be perfectly legitimate, even if it was spent in the course of a second marriage. Some people certainly will try to preserve assets for their own children (as in the case of Sandra Thompson and Paul Watson quoted above), but there is no moral requirement to do so. Especially when such situations are viewed from the child's perspective, most people indicate that they are happy for their parents to spend money while they are alive. The fact that a step-parent will also benefit from this does not cause concern. For example, Patricia Lacey, speaking of her father, who divorced her mother, married again and subsequently died, indicates that she was quite happy to have received nothing from her father's estate:

INTERVIEWER: Did you know that it was all going to his second wife?
PATRICIA: Oh yes.
INTERVIEWER: He actually said that to you?
PATRICIA: Well no. But I mean I knew. He's not exactly a millionaire. He was just an average man, you know ... They didn't have their pockets lined with gold or anything. I didn't expect to get anything, and I wasn't disappointed when I didn't.

(Patricia Lacey, under 40, married, home owner)

Her step-mother did receive something when her father died. But Patricia is quite comfortable about that because she knew that her father 'was just an average man ... didn't have [his] pockets lined with gold'. She displays no sense that her father had an obligation to conserve resources in order to leave them to her.

So children in complex families do not have the right to expect their parents to provide for them through inheritance. *If there is anything left*, then it should go to the children rather than fall into someone else's hands. This point is expressed neatly in our interview with Madonna Smith, who was divorced and cohabiting with another partner at the time we interviewed her. She had entered into a complicated series of property deals since beginning to live with her new partner, partly to try to maximise their assets and partly to enable them ultimately to live in a more suitable house than either previously owned. At the time of the interview, she and her partner owned three houses between them, two of them being rented to students, at least on a temporary basis. Her partner Tony owned the least valuable of the three houses because Madonna, as she put it, 'had a thirteen-year head start on him' in the property market. Their ultimate aim was to have one house for their own use, which Madonna would own, and one to rent out as a source of income, which Tony would own. Madonna was clear that she would never own a house jointly with Tony because of the disparity of their positions in the housing market ('We haven't actually bought anything between us, and wouldn't').

Madonna was aware that between them their assets were substantial ('you are talking about over a quarter of a million'). She had therefore made a will in favour of her own children from her previous marriage. Her motivation, however, was not so much to secure her children's future as to deprive her ex-husband of any possible benefit:

> I did this will because, with us, it isn't actually who we want to have it. It's who we don't want to have it (laughs). I mean I don't want my ex-husband walking in here and taking everything, and what have you, because he is the father of the children.
> (Madonna Smith, 40s, divorced and cohabiting, first-generation home owner)

In this comment, Madonna pinpoints the emotional bite of our narrative: you don't want money to fall into the wrong hands ('It isn't who we want to have it. It's who we *don't want* to have it'). What most troubles her is not the thought of having nothing to leave to her children but the thought that she might have something to leave but that her ex-husband might take it. She is making a very important and much more general point here: that a testator should be able to *choose* who should have their money, and who should not.

Children and step-children

These interviews provide data not simply on the circumstances in which children and step-children inherit but on how people approach the *division of assets between individuals*.

In Chapter 3, we consider the more general question of how assets are or should be divided between children. We show there that the principle of *equal treatment* emerges as the starting point for most people's thinking about how to divide their assets between individuals. However, this is not always a straightforward matter, even in families where there has been no history of divorce or remarriage. Complex families pose even bigger challenges.

We begin exploring those challenges by looking first at situations where there are no step-children but an individual has children from different relationships. Although at first sight this may seem relatively straightforward, in reality it is not, at least in some cases. The very fact that there has been a divorce means that there are, at least in principle, two estates rather than one in which children have an interest. If further children are then born, to different marriages (or marriage-like relationships), the situation can become very complex because different children have different combinations of parents from whom they may or may not inherit. If an individual parent is attempting to ensure that all his or her children get treated equally in relation to inheritance, the problem is *not* the principle of equal treatment. It is working out *how to apply* that principle.

We can explore these complexities through the case of Phoebe Rogers, aged 42 when we interviewed her and living alone. Her history of marriage and cohabitation runs like this:

- Had a child when she was 17; was not married. The child was given up for adoption, and she has had no further contact.
- Married for six months in her early 20s; no children.
- Cohabitation for two to three years; a son.
- Cohabitation for approximately five years; a daughter.
- Living alone.

Phoebe thus has two children, each with a different father, both born in cohabiting relationships that have now ended. Both her former cohabitees, and indeed her ex-husband, now have new partners. The history of property ownership within these sets of relationships causes Phoebe considerable concern, because she feels that, on each occasion, she brought more resources to the relationship than did her partners, but that each of them benefited when assets were divided after the relationship had ended. She therefore feels keenly the inheritance position of her son and her daughter. Her calculations about this depend on the commitments of her ex-partners that arise from other liaisons. It is necessary to give quite a lengthy quote here in order to bring out the nuances:

PHOEBE: It's nice this idea of leaving something to my children. I'd like to see that they're well cared for. My daughter I'm less worried about ... My son's father has made a will and left everything to his wife. And when he dies, my son gets a sixth of whatever's left. Because my son's father actually spawned children all over the place (laughter). He's got quite a lot of children – I think about five that he actually sees. I think probably there are more.
INTERVIEWER: Right.

PHOEBE: So he's got one in Australia as well as my son. He's got two daughters over here. So that's – one, two, three, four. Oh! – perhaps it's that my son gets a sixth – hang on. I think when his wife dies, most of it goes to his son in Australia and the rest of it goes between the other children. So he'll probably get half and the other three will get a third, will get a sixth each.

INTERVIEWER: You've actually talked to him about inheritance for your son?

PHOEBE: I haven't talked to his father. My son's told me this. His father wrote to him and told him what he'd put in his will. My daughter's father was running a business and bought himself a beautiful Georgian house out at Fullton, with barns where he was running his business which he bought with his girlfriend. And her three children moved in and then they split up. And then he had to buy her out, and then he just lost his business, lost everything. He's now living in rented accommodation. So where he was full of 'What I'm going to leave my children' – he's a son by a previous marriage ... He's got absolutely zilch ... I actually felt at one point, my kids will always be OK because they've got two dads who seem to be doing all right, and are going to provide partly for them. And then with what I have as well, they don't seem to be doing too badly. But I think things have changed over the last couple of years (laughter) ...

INTERVIEWER: So your daughter presumably would have been getting quite a bit more than your son?

PHOEBE: Than my son – yes.

INTERVIEWER: Would you have taken that into account when you wrote your will, do you think?

PHOEBE: Yes. But my daughter's terribly mercenary (laughter).

(Phoebe Rogers, 40s, divorced, home owner)

What Phoebe shows in this extract is an acute sense of the different positions of each of her children. In order to keep this up to date, she has made sure that she knows the financial situations of her former partners with a reasonable degree of precision – largely it would seem through information provided by her children. She had previously judged that her daughter stood to inherit considerably more from her father than her son did from his father, although she believes that recently her daughter's father has lost most of his money following the break-up of his subsequent relationship. The situation with her daughter is clearly volatile, and she is trying to keep abreast of this. Her son's position seems to be more predictable in that his father has made a will and has written to him to tell him what proportion he will receive. It will not be much, however, since her son's father has a total of five children with a variety of partners ('he has spawned children all over the place'). Her own motivation for keeping up to date with the financial circumstances of her former partners is partly to enable her to take decisions about the disposition of her own property. She indicates that if her daughter were indeed to get more than her son from their respective fathers, then she would consider redressing that balance through her own will. She also indicates that, were she able to trace the son she gave up for adoption, she would also like to leave him something, although it might be just 'a nominal amount'.

This case shows us not merely how serial relationships (in this case, without marriage, but that does not alter the fundamental issue) put an individual's children in very different positions in respect of inheritance, even when no step-children are involved. The principle of equal treatment cannot be applied straightforwardly if one wishes to achieve *equality of outcome*, that is where all children end up with the same resources through inheritance. However, trying to achieve equality of outcome may be extremely difficult without full knowledge of what the other parent is going to do. It also means that your own children may have to be treated *unequally* in order to achieve the desired outcome – a gesture that runs the risk of being misunderstood.

When step-children enter the picture, the same issues can arise in an even more complex form. In Variation 2 of our narrative we indicated that, according to our interviewees, it is quite acceptable for step-children to inherit under certain circumstances. We have also noted that our wills data show cases where step-children inherit in a way that appears to treat them as more analogous to children than to any other category of kin. We now look more closely at the circumstances under which step-children do inherit from step-parents, and how they are treated by comparison with children who have the genetic link.

It is clear from our data that the simple fact of being a stepchild does not tell us anything about whether that person is likely to be a beneficiary of the step-parent's estate. We know from our wills data, reported above, that *some* step-children seem to be treated on the same basis as children, while others are not; but with very small numbers of step-children mentioned at all it is difficult to draw any further conclusions from the wills sample. Our interview study gives us a better feel for this, but our interviewees were not chosen randomly and therefore we cannot use this as the basis for generalising to the whole population of step-families.

Nonetheless, our interviews do indicate that there is no single way in which step-relationships are handled when it comes to determining inheritance. In our study population, we had nine individuals who were step-parents, fourteen whose own children were step-children (because they had themselves formed a new relationship) and twelve people who were themselves, or had been, step-children. Because some people fall into more than one of these categories, a total of twenty-seven interviewees thus had some direct experience of step-families.

We probed the inheritance experience and intentions of interviewees in all these categories but found no consistent pattern. Of the nine who themselves had step-children, two had not decided what to do about inheritance; three wanted to bequeath to their step-children on precisely the same terms as their genetic children; and four were distinguishing between their children and step-children in a variety of ways. There was a similar variety when we asked people about what inheritance they had received from a deceased step-parent, and what they expected to receive from a living one, except that some people in this group said that they had received – or expected to receive – nothing because the step-parent had nothing to bequeath.

Putting this together with the wills data, it seems fairly clear that some step-children are treated as 'full children' when it comes to inheritance, while others are not. However, even when they are not, this does not necessarily mean that step-children are discriminated against or treated as less important. One characteristic of step-families is that different children have different combinations of parents and are therefore likely to inherit from different sources, at different points in time. If one takes a snapshot by interviewing just one of those parents, the picture has to be interpreted carefully. Take for example Isle Whittaker, a woman in her sixties who had been married, divorced, remarried and widowed. She had two children from her first marriage and a step-daughter from her second. She had written her will and had left her estate to be divided between the three of them. However, her step-daughter would receive a smaller proportion than her own two children because, as Isle saw it, the step-daughter had already inherited a substantial amount from her father (Isle's second husband) when he died. She felt that the relationship directly between her and her step-daughter should properly result in a bequest from her, but that she owed her less than she did her own children. This example illustrates the importance of understanding the snapshot picture (in this case, Isle's own bequeathing intentions) with reference to the moving picture of family life as it evolves over time.

With due caution, therefore, can we pinpoint any reason why some step-children seem to be treated as 'full children' for inheritance purposes, while others are not? The most obvious single reason derives from the circumstances under which the relationship with the step-child was formed. To take the most obvious cases, where a step-child was young at the time of the second marriage and was, at least in part, brought up by the step-parent, these are circumstances under which people seem to sanction treating step-children as 'full children'. One such case is described to us by Mollie Avenham, who had remarried when her youngest child was still quite small. He was brought up in the household with her second husband, who clearly grew to be very fond of him. Her husband is now dead, but Mollie reports this about his intentions concerning inheritance at a time when her son was young:

MOLLIE: So we both made a will at that time [i.e. when they married]. Because he never had any children and Barry was a little boy, the son he would love to have had. And he wanted his property to be left to Barry. Barry loved that house, you know. And I made my will that the other house in Maple Street, at the bottom end of town, was sold and divided between the three children. And of course three years after my second husband died. So then I made another will.
INTERVIEWER: And Barry would be – he was still at school? Just a little boy.
MOLLIE: Well I think he would be about eleven.
INTERVIEWER: How did you feel about him wanting that property to go to Barry and not to the other two?

MOLLIE: Well we agreed on that when we sold the two houses. You know, he was quite happy with that. And I felt it was fair.
(Mollie Avenham, 70s, divorced, currently in local authority rented accommodation, having previously been a home owner)

Mollie's husband wrote a will that made her youngest son Barry his main beneficiary, whereas her own will treated all her three children equally. The reasons she gives for this are that Barry was 'just a little boy' (by implication in need of more support than the two older children, who had already left home) and that her husband was particularly fond of Barry ('the son he would have loved to have'). The implication of both is that the role of *actively parenting* a young child creates bonds between two individuals that the step-parent understandably wants to acknowledge through inheritance, as in other ways.

Mollie's daughter, Sandra Fisher, provides a case that illustrates the same point in a rather different way. It is the second marriage for both Sandra and her husband, and they have jointly brought up two children, one from each of their first marriages. Meanwhile, in both cases their former spouse has remarried and had another child. The interview discusses the question of inheritance coming from various different parents in these terms:

INTERVIEWER: Do you know if [your ex-husband] has written a will?
SANDRA: I don't think so. He's since had another child.
INTERVIEWER: Oh he's remarried, has he?
SANDRA: Yes. So I think it's possible that the child would inherit.
INTERVIEWER: And what about your husband? Has [his ex-wife] remarried?
SANDRA: Yes she has.
INTERVIEWER: And has she got more children now?
SANDRA: Yes she's got one. So I presume the same would happen.
INTERVIEWER: You think the same would happen – that the other two wouldn't really get anything from that side of the family?
SANDRA: No. I think – because we've had them for all these years and we've taken the responsibility. So it's up to us to leave them sorted out.
(Sandra Fisher, 40s, second marriage, home owner)

This extract from Sandra's interview is very interesting because she makes it clear, first that her initial reaction is that the younger children, the children of subsequent marriages, would automatically take precedence. However, when pressed, the issue is not really about favouring the children of the extant marriage. It is actually an issue of the person who 'takes responsibility' for bringing up a child also thereby accepts the responsibility to 'leave them sorted out'. Thus where a step-parent and step-child have formed a close personal relationship – 'bringing up' being the most obvious circumstance where it is likely to happen – it does introduce a new principle to set alongside the importance of the genetic link.

The possibility not only of including step-children as well as children but also of distinguishing between one step-child and another when it comes to inheritance opens up the possibility of very delicate calculations about the terms on which each individual should be treated. We can now return to our discussion of *the principle of equal treatment*, but this time including step-children in the picture. We do this through an exploration of the family circumstances of Mavis and Ken Douglas. The reason for selecting the Douglas case in the context of this discussion is that this couple has two 'shared' children and also one surviving child from Mavis' first marriage. So they offer an example of how people try to divide their assets in a 'mixed' family. The discussion is particularly striking because Ken in particular had not thought, before the interview, of the possibility of his step-daughter inheriting from her genetic father. Thus in the interview itself, we see how he tries to think it through.

The family discussed below includes:

- Mavis and Ken Douglas, married with three adult children. Second marriage for Mavis, first for Ken. Both aged 54.
- Mavis' children from her first marriage.
- Julie, aged 31. Married with children aged 8, 6 and 4.
- Wayne (deceased). Would have been 29. Killed in a car accident at the age of 18. Mavis separated from her first husband when Wayne was six months old.
- Ken's and Mavis' children:
- Jason. Aged 22. Has just joined the armed forces.
- Kate. Aged 20. Still living in the parental home.

Mavis and Ken own their own home, as did both their respective parents, and they have made wills. We have a detailed account from them about how their thinking operated in the division of their estate between their children, of whom there were four at the time when they first made wills. Mavis says that they were 'advised' to make wills many years ago because they had a family that included step-children ('even though we don't call them step-children'). Ken says that they first decided to make wills because it seemed the 'sensible' thing to do (a phrase that he uses several times). His emphasis is on the number of children rather than the fact that they include step-children:

> It seemed a sensible thing to do, when there were four of them, to make sure that everybody got a little bit of something, you know.
> (Ken Douglas, 50s, married, home owner)

In terms of the content of the wills, Mavis describes hers as

> a very simple one. It's just divided equally, with jewellery going to certain ones.
> (Mavis Douglas, 50s, second marriage, home owner)

Ken confirms that his will is in the same format. The advice (from a solicitor, who is also described as a friend) was to divide everything equally between the four children. The wills had to be remade when Wayne was killed, but the same principle of equal division was retained.

Mavis and Ken are clearly operating the principle that all their children should be treated equally, without reference to who the father is. In introducing this issue, Mavis says:

> We were advised to split it equally so that there wasn't any animosity about anything, if anything happened. There was nothing really to think about. Because the children are all like Ken's children anyway. I mean anyone coming into the home would never know that they weren't all his children. They were all treated the same. That's how we always wanted it.

Again we see that the issue of bringing up children comes into play ('anyone coming into the home would never know that they weren't all [Ken's] children'). Ken says less about how the principle of equality was arrived at but treats it as more of a moral as well as a practical issue ('the right way to do it'; 'you have to have peace of mind that it will be done properly'):

> It seemed a sensible thing to do when there were four of them, to make sure that everybody got a little bit of something, you know. And I think that's the right way to do it ... I think it was the sensible thing to do to be honest. I think so. You have, somehow you have to have a peace of mind that it will be done properly don't you?
> (Ken Douglas, 50s, married, home owner)

So far it seems simple, a straightforward example of treating stepchildren as 'full children'. However, what about equality of outcome? As we have shown, other interviewees think of equality of outcome, not equality of division, when they talk about treating children equally. Is this an issue in the Douglas family? During the course of the interview, it became clear that the possibility of inequalities being introduced through one child's inheriting from her genetic father seems to be something that neither has ever thought of. When faced with the question, the reactions of Ken and Mavis are different.

Mavis, when the possibility is put to her, says that it has not affected her thinking *and would not do so*. She immediately evokes the principle that all her children should be entitled to *equal shares from her*. Presumably this means that what any of them gets from someone else is not relevant to the principle of equality, as she sees it.

INTERVIEWER: If you thought that they would inherit some money from their father, do you think that would have altered how you wrote your will?
MAVIS: No! No! Not at all. It didn't have any bearing on it at all. But I don't think there's any danger of that (laughs).
INTERVIEWER: Right. Why wouldn't you take it into consideration then?
MAVIS: Because Julie and Wayne are just as much mine as Jason and Kate. So I would think they would be entitled to as much

of mine as they ... And they were. No I don't think – I just wouldn't alter it at all.

(Mavis Douglas, 50s, second marriage, home owner)

By contrast, Ken's reaction to the suggestion about Julie inheriting from her genetic father is one of real astonishment:

INTERVIEWER: Do you anticipate that Julie might get anything from your wife's first husband? In terms of inheritance?
KEN: Gosh! I've never even thought about that. Gosh yes. What a thought!
INTERVIEWER: It's not something that's ever?
KEN: I've never, I've never even contemplated it. We've been a fairly tightly knit complete family really, you know. And that's just never entered my head at all.

(Ken Douglas, 50s, married, home owner)

The interviewer then presses him to consider whether he would change his own will if he thought that Julie was going to inherit from her genetic father. Like Mavis, he says that it would make no difference, but the context in which he sees that is slightly different from hers:

INTERVIEWER: Do you think, if you were to expect Julie to have some money from her father, you would take that into consideration?
KEN: No.
INTERVIEWER: No? You'd still write the same will?
KEN: Right. Because hopefully she would, if there was anything like that, I'm sure she would do the right thing by the others anyway. I would have thought. That is something I've never seriously contemplated.
INTERVIEWER: In the sense of giving a bit more back to them, do you mean to do the right thing?
KEN: No. From, that Julie would, perhaps pass on some to the others. That's what I meant.
INTERVIEWER: To her brothers and sisters?
KEN: Yes.

(Ken Douglas, 50s, married, home owner)

Ken's reaction is similar to Mavis' in that he sticks by the principle that all the children should inherit equally from him. By implication, to do anything else would be to deny that they have always been a 'tightly knit complete family'.

However, unlike Mavis, he does see the possibility of Julie's inheriting from her genetic father as a problem in that it would create inequities within the sibling group. Ken's instincts are that the children should receive bequests in such a way that *there is equality of outcome*. Thinking out loud in the interview, he reasons with himself that the only way to resolve this would be for Julie herself to take the initiative and pass on some of her 'extra' inheritance to her siblings. The concept of equality between the siblings is thus his paramount consideration. Given that he had not thought of this possibility previously, his only solution is to rely on Julie to 'do the right thing by the others'.

In these extracts, we see a married couple trying to think through in practical terms how to treat their own children so as to achieve the desired outcome. We also see that they are thinking this through against the backdrop of cultural meaning and values that their situation evokes. Ken's desire to have 'peace of mind that it will be done properly' shows that he is aware of this. His own personal wishes are shaped against a background that there is a 'proper' way of doing things, for which there is an audience both inside and outside the family. Mavis is equally aware of this audience, but in a different way. She is conscious that a differential division of her own estate could be misinterpreted as undervaluing the children from her first marriage. She describes them as 'just as much mine' as the younger two.

There is therefore a good deal at stake in the handling of inheritance from a parent's perspective, and this is made particularly tricky in complex families. The stakes are high because the way in which assets are distributed – and perhaps more importantly the way in which others interpret this distribution – makes a public statement about the way in which a parent values each of her or his children.

Types of property

So far we have referred simply to 'inheritance' without discussion of *what* is passed on. However, it will be apparent that, for many people, the 'what' is not particularly important. From our analysis of 800 wills, we see that about half the testators make no distinction at all between different types of property, rolling it into a single 'estate' that is then distributed in proportions to the beneficiaries. Most of the rest make a few specific bequests before rolling the rest together (see Chapter 3 for a fuller discussion of this). The small number of wills where we know there is a complex family (that is, where step-children are mentioned) follow the general pattern.

Turning to the interview study, it will be apparent from the examples used so far that most people are not concerned to preserve specific items of property for their children but that they have the rather more nebulous concern that children should get 'something'. It must be acknowledged that our study deliberately focused upon ordinary families, not those who are wealthy or landed, where we might have found a greater concern with the specifics of individual items of property. But in the 'ordinary' families that we studied, this seems not to be the case except in those examples where an interviewee is talking about the possibility of a parent's dying when the child is still young. In these cases, there is a specific concern about what will happen to the *house*. This clearly reflects the need to ensure that, in such circumstances, a child continues to have a home in which he or she has the right to live and access to the resources to maintain until attaining adulthood.

This consideration is obviously particularly pertinent in complex families, because normally children live with only one of their genetic parents. If that parent has not acquired a new partner, the prospect of their death potentially removes the child's home in a way that does not happen if there are two resident parents. If the resident parent does have a new partner, the situation is more ambiguous than in first marriages, in terms of ownership of the property and responsibility for providing the children with a home. Thus we see Angela Sale (quoted above) insisting that her home is for her children, not for her cohabitee, even though she would be happy for him to live there temporarily and bring them up.

Angela had not actually made provision through a will for this outcome, but others in similar circumstances have done so. For example, Jane Clark, a woman in her twenties, told us that she had done precisely this. Jane was married at the time of her interview but had a child from a previous relationship with a man to whom she was not married. She told us that while she was cohabiting with her previous partner she had bought a house and that when the relationship ended she wanted to ensure that her son's rights to inherit it would be preserved. She said:

> Me and James' Dad split up a couple of years ago, and we weren't married, and there was a lot of legal hassles as you can imagine when you split up, with a child. So I wrote a will leaving the house, the money everything to James and [I wrote] that my Mum should look after him, that he should be sent to my Mum's to live, if anything ever happened to me.
> (Jane Clark, 20s, married, home owner)

The particular arrangement that she favoured was to leave all her assets to her child but to make her mother the child's guardian on the assumption that he would actually go to live with his grandmother. This will was written after Jane had split from her previous partner. She has subsequently married, but she has not changed the will. She insists that 'the will still stands even though I've married Geoff', although she admits that she does not know whether being married will 'change any legalities over the will'. But her intentions are clear. She remains the owner of the house in which she lives with her husband and son. Should she die, she would like the house to go to her son in order to ensure that he continues to have a home. In practical terms, she thinks that he might still go to live with her mother ('he'd probably be better off with my Mum. She's got more patience with him than anyone else'). But the point is that the house remains *hers* because she feels that her first responsibility is to provide her son with a home. She says that 'eventually ... the house will go into mine and Geoff's names', but she is in no hurry to put the principle of joint ownership into effect.

Interestingly, Jane has not actually discussed any of this with her husband. Unlike some other families (for example, the Douglas family quoted above), who want a step-parent to become a 'real parent' as rapidly as possible, Jane and some other people in this situation believe that they themselves retain full responsibility for providing for the child of a previous marriage or relationship. Hence the focus on providing a home for the child after one dies. If she is going to fall back on anyone, it will be her mother: 'I will leave it all in her capable hands (laughs). That's what mothers are for, isn't it?'

Her mother, Julie Hilton, whom we also interviewed, echoed Jane's view by telling us that although she feels no particular obligation to provide an inheritance for her children and intended to spend up before she dies, she does feel that she should make some special provision for James at the moment because 'he's more like a child than a grandchild'. Although neither she nor her husband Roy has made a will, if they get round to doing so she feels that she should leave something 'in trust' for James because 'he's very young, he's only three'.

Houses therefore have a particular resonance in our data about providing for young children because they represent the parent's continuing commitment to provide a home. That commitment is a personal rather than a shared one where divorce has ensured that a child has only one resident genetic parent. Although some people treat step-parents as 'replacement parents' in this regard, this is not true of all our interviewees, some of whom retain clear personal responsibility and, if they need fall back, it is to the child's grandparents (who do have the genetic link) rather than their new partner.

Apart from mentioning houses in these specific circumstances, the other type of property that our interviewees talk about is *jewellery*, or sometimes other small personal items. In some of these examples, we do see the importance of the genetic link emerging even in families where they are at pains to treat children and step-children on the same terms. A good example is offered by Mavis and Ken Douglas, whose situation we discussed above as an example of a couple who strive to make no distinction between children and step-children. However, when it comes to jewellery a slightly different message emerges. Mavis speaks about a ring that she was given by Ken's mother and specifies that this will go to Kate, her younger daughter, because she is the 'natural grandchild' of her mother-in-law:

MAVIS: Like that ring which my mother-in-law gave me will go to Kate, my youngest daughter, because she is her natural grandchild, rather than to Julie the eldest daughter – which it would normally do, wouldn't it?
INTERVIEWER: What made you decide that you wanted to say that the ring was going ...

MAVIS: Because I felt it was right. I felt it was Kate's right, that the ring went to her. Because it was her grandmother's. And my other jewellery went to Julie, the eldest one.

(Mavis Douglas, 50s, second marriage, home owner)

So, despite the fact that Mavis and Ken do not like to use the term 'step-children' (see above), and they want to treat them all equally, the genetic link does matter when it comes to these specific items. However, Mavis also still tries to ensure that her younger daughter is not thereby advantaged by saying that her elder daughter will get her own jewellery – a kind of 'balancing' bequest – but of course there is a genetic link there also.

Thus, in complex families, we see an interplay between step-relationships and genetic relationships when it comes to inheritance, with the significance of the 'blood line' apparently coming into play where there is property with *symbolic* significance, like jewellery, even if the principle of equal treatment of children and step-children is being applied. However, this principle is not always applied. It is particularly likely to occur in circumstances where step-parent and step-child have formed a close personal relationship, often but not necessarily when the child was young. Thus step-children are seen as legitimate people to inherit property but not to the exclusion of children who have the genetic link. If the parent does leave an estate, then genetic children should get a reasonable proportion of it and should be the ones who inherit those personal items that are the most symbolically significant.

Conclusion: family and kinship

In this final section, we want to draw out what our analysis of inheritance in complex families tells us about the nature of family and kinship in contemporary English society. This also points the way forward to some of the major themes that are developed in subsequent chapters.

The starting point for this book was a set of theoretical debates about the nature of kinship in the English context, in which the concept of individualism has been central. At its simplest level, this means that there is presumed to be a *flexibility* about both kinship structures and the expectations associated with them. It is of particular interest when we look at family and kinship in complex families. By definition, these are families whose structure has been modified through some combination of divorce, remarriage, the birth of 'sets' of children who have different combinations of parents, and the creation of step-relationships. The way in which such families handle inheritance issues enables us to see how they define and redefine kinship in the process of managing these changes.

Our central conclusion is that people take full advantage of the openness of English inheritance law to make their own choices about how to redefine 'my family' as they move through the changes associated with divorce, separation, repartnering and step-relationships. Some would appear to stay with a fairly simple definition focused on the line of descent and its genetic links. Examples used in this chapter would include Angela Sale and Jane Clark, each of whom has taken advantage of their ability under English law both to own property and to decide to whom they will pass it on. Each of them sees her children as her heirs and is explicitly by-passing her current partner (despite the fact that in general there is a presumption that a surviving spouse inherits). Although Angela is cohabiting, Jane is actually married to her current partner. But she still sees her core family as constituting herself, her son and her mother for all significant purposes. However, once in a new partnership, other people define their core family as the new partner plus all the children associated with one or both of them. Mavis and Ken Douglas, Mollie Avenham and Sandra Fisher are all cases used in this chapter that illustrate this alternative model.

Thus we see that there is a *selection process* at work in determining how an individual's kin group is constituted for inheritance purposes. There is a freedom of choice, which people do exercise to suit their own circumstances, about the terms on which individuals are included. This is not so much about who 'counts' as kin but about the commitments associated with each relationship, and especially about who is treated as a member of the most intimate family circle. 'Biological' children are almost always included. A current spouse is also automatically included, but with some conditions attached if it is a second or subsequent marriage, where the nature of the commitment to a second spouse is limited by the need to acknowledge commitments to children. Stepchildren may also be included as members of the family on the same terms as children, although they need not be. Thus we see that the selection process works *within a defined range*, which does have boundaries.

Being able to define one's family *according to circumstances* is in fact a key feature of English kinship as seen through the lens of inheritance. This allows for people to adapt, and perhaps more importantly *to go on adapting*, their definition of who constitutes 'my family' as they move through life. Thus we see that it is possible to make a distinction between first and second marriages, and the expectations associated with them, precisely because the circumstances in which they occur are not the same. It is also possible to make changes in the way that assets are divided between children and step-children, depending on circumstances prevailing at a given time, including knowledge about what an individual will receive from the other parent.

All this fits well with our suggestions in Chapter 1 that English kinship is based on 'persons' more than genealogical positions, and on practices of reflexive relationism. The kin networks of any one individual are clearly constituted, and reconstituted over time, through their relationships. Personal choice and the quality of relationships play an important and accepted role in who is included. The core with which people work out how to treat children and step-children on equitable terms reinforces the importance of these choices. There are no discernible differences between women and men in the matter of property transmission. Complex families display these opportunities very visibly. However, they also apparently display some elements of fixity, which is a thread running through this highly flexible, distinctively English, approach to kinship.

The core thread of fixity is the continuing relationship between parents and children. This remains at the core even in complex families, where people's definition of 'my family' can be highly personal. But the parent–child relationship is both predictable and privileged, as is seen very clearly in relation to inheritance. The central imagery of inheritance in these complex families – that money should not 'pass out of the family' – is actually a moral statement that the privileged relationship between parent and child should be reconfirmed at the end of the parent's life. It is the position of children that must be confirmed, not 'the family' more generally, and this demonstrates that there are very strong links between inheritance and *active parenting*.

However, what of the concept of family property? We argued in Chapter 1 that individualist or ego-focused kinship systems are characterised by a weak sense of 'family property'; no real sense of a common stake in resources across the generations or that one generation holds property 'in trust' for the next. But our case study of inheritance in complex families throws up some paradoxes in relation to a family stake in property. The core theme of our inheritance narrative – that money should not pass out of the family – appears to make a strong statement about a common stake.

Under the surface, however, the message is slightly different. First, the emphasis on transmission down the generations is modified by a universal acceptance that a surviving spouse inherits everything. There may be some moral restrictions where, in the context of a second marriage, there is clear disparity in what resources each partner 'brought in', but essentially children do not have claims while there is a living step-parent.

Second, children do not have a right to expect inheritance, and parents do not have a responsibility to leave any assets. They can spend everything during their lifetime if they so choose, and that expenditure can be shared with a second or subsequent spouse. In this sense, there is a very weak common stake in property across the generations. The principle that the parent–child link must be confirmed through inheritance only comes into play *if* there are assets to bequeath. In those circumstances, the position of children is guarded jealously, particularly against the possibility that resources might pass to someone with only a distant connection through second marriage. The real emotion in this narrative is generated by that possibility. It is not merely that children lose out. It is also that resources pass to someone who has no real connection, either genetic or personal, and who has not been, nor would have been, *chosen* by the testator.

Thus the principle of a common stake in property across the generations comes into play only in special circumstances: where there is no surviving spouse; where a parent has left assets to bequeath rather than using them all; and where the deceased parent has made no explicit choices (either in a will or otherwise) about the distribution of her or his property. In these circumstances, there is a strongly felt belief that resources should not simply drift away by default, and the claims of children are asserted.

Our case study of complex families therefore opens up questions about the nature of English kinship, which we explore in subsequent chapters through our data on a broader range of family circumstances, including many where there has been no history of remarriage or step-relationships. The case of families with experience of divorce, separation, repartnering and step-relationships demonstrates what variety is permitted and accepted within English kinship. It tells us less about what constitutes the norm. We now turn to this broader picture.

Chapter 3

Transmissions and divisions

Introduction: the transmission of property

In this chapter, we move from a specific case study of families with experience of divorce, separation, repartnering and step-relationships (developed in Chapter 2) to providing an outline map of the 'big picture'. The chapter is centred on the fundamental concept of property and its transmission from one person to another through inheritance. Through this, we shall consider what the process of passing on property tells us about the way in which family and kinship are understood and lived.

To set the scene for this discussion, the first step is to sketch out how property is transmitted. We consider both the mechanisms that are available to allow an individual to pass on property after his or her death, and also which mechanisms are important in practice. We are concentrating in this chapter on transmission following a death, but it is always open to anyone to give away property during their lifetime. Our interview data do contain some examples of lifetime transfers, and we refer to these in later chapters, but for the most part our analysis centres on transmissions that follow a death. Under English law, property can be transmitted after a person's death in one of three ways: through administration of small estates without recourse to a will, through a will or via intestacy legislation (Finch *et al.* 1996).

It is well known that only a minority of the English population does exercise the right to make a will, currently around one-third (Finch *et al.* 1996). On the face of it, this seems curious in a legal system that leaves the choice of beneficiary so open-ended. However, our interview data indicate that a number of people who do not write wills believe that it is unnecessary for them to do so because intestacy legislation will produce the outcome they want in any event. There is a belief that property will pass to a spouse or children 'automatically', and therefore there is no need to write a will if that is the outcome one desires. However, many interviewees have a very hazy idea of what the legislation actually is, and the solicitors we interviewed warned against the assumption that intestacy legislation will straightforwardly produce the desired outcome.

Our own study of 800 wills tells us something about the composition of the population of people who do make a will, although it can only tell us about 'last' wills – that is, the will valid when a person dies (see Finch *et al.* 1996 for a full review of this study). These data show that roughly equal numbers of women and men have made a will by the time they die. They also tell us that 'last' wills are likely to be made in old age. The median age at which the 'last' will is written is 69 (men) and 73 (women). Around half of the wills were written between the ages of 61 and 77 (for men) and 65 and 81 (for women). There is a strong sense of the final settlement of one's affairs coming through in this sample of wills. This seems to be the dominant pattern. However, there certainly are people who write a will at a younger age, when their life circumstances could be very different from those at the time of their death but who nonetheless allow that early will to stand – 25 per cent of the wills in our sample were written ten years before the testator died.

There is no way of knowing how many of these last wills are also first wills – that is, the only one ever made. If that were the case, then we could deduce that most people only think about making a will as they get older and, presumably, as the prospect of their own death becomes more real. The wills data cannot give us access to that information. However, we can learn something more about that issue by comparing the wills study with our interview data. This enables us to see at a more individual level what prompts people to write a will. Although this was not designed as a representative sample, it did cover people of a wide range of ages, living in a variety of social and economic circumstances. We selected our interviewees to cover a range of 'ordinary' families. Although we cannot make formal generalisations about will makers on the basis of this group, we have no reason to suppose that they are a notably unrepresentative group except in one respect, namely that we deliberately included a high proportion of home owners, who represent three-quarters of our study population.

A total of forty people told us that they had already written a will. This represents thirty-six of our 'cases', since four were from joint interviews with married couples. Thus just under half (41 per cent) of our interviewees had made a will, a slightly higher proportion than in the general population. In this mixed-age study population, women are a little more likely to have written a will than men, but gender is not a major factor distinguishing between those who have made a will and those who have not.

Of particular relevance to the present study is the question of whether home ownership prompts people to write a will. One reason for undertaking this study is that we were conscious of the major social changes under way in British society as a consequence of the spread of home ownership (see Chapter 1). We reasoned that, for large numbers of people, they would be the first generation in their own families with something significant to bequeath, and we wondered what differences this might make to their approach to questions of inheritance within their own families. We deliberately included a majority of the study population as home owners, with a proportion of them being the first generation in their own families to own a house.

In fact, housing tenure is not the distinguishing factor that explains which people have made a will. Of the seventy-six home owners in the study, thirty-one reported that they had made a will (41 per cent). This compares with nine of our twenty-two non-home owners (also 41 percent). There are some differences according to whether a person's parents also owned their own home, which we discuss in Chapter 5, but the simple distinction between being a home owner and not does not explain patterns of will making.

By far the most important factor in predicting whether one of our study population has made a will is age. People over 60 are very likely to have done so. For those under 60 it is much less predictable. In our interview study, forty individuals had made wills, twenty-five of whom were over 60. Indeed, almost all the over sixties in the study had made a will (only two had not), whereas only one-fifth of interviewees under 60 had done so.

In those relatively unusual cases where younger people have made a will, there is a certain predictability about their reasons for doing so, as reported to us. If we take the eleven people under 50 who had made a will (nine of whom were women), their reasons fall essentially into two categories: divorce and travel. In the first category, we find some people whose own divorce (or the breakdown of a cohabiting relationship) had prompted them to make a will to ensure that their children received their property. This is very much in line with what we were told in our interviews with solicitors, many of whom said that they felt it to be their professional duty to advise divorcing couples to make wills. This advice may not always be followed, however; certainly, some divorcees in our study population had not made a will.

The prospect of travel was the factor most commonly mentioned by these younger interviewees in explaining why they had written a will. Mainly it was travel that appeared to carry the possibility of a dramatic death – the first experience of flying in an aeroplane, long-distance driving with all members of the family in the same car, a trip to a distant part of the world. These seem to be events that give some reality to the possibility of one's own death, which otherwise appears insufficiently real to most younger people to lead them to take steps that anticipate its consequences.

Wills are only one way in which property may be distributed after a person dies. Our data suggest that they are of relatively limited importance in the sense that much property passes by other means: through joint ownership between spouses; through legislation that provides for the administration of small estates without recourse to a will; through intestacy rules; through direct gifts by the testator before he or she dies; and through agreement between beneficiaries, who decide on the detailed distribution of property after a death. Indeed, our interviews suggest that these mechanisms for reaching informal agreement are widely assumed to be the desirable way of proceeding in families and are a touchstone for demonstrating that the family works well because it does not need to have recourse to the law to settle its affairs. The following quote is fairly typical of this perspective. It comes from Mavis Douglas, a woman in her fifties who had been married twice and who had children from both marriages. Despite the fairly complex calculations about the claims of different children on major assets (see the analysis of the Douglas case in Chapter 2), when it comes to items of personal and household property Mavis expects her children to decide on the distribution informally.

MAVIS: They all get on very, very well. They are all friends. I don't think there'd be any trouble, you know. They'd just take what they wanted, I suppose. I've not sort of said 'That picture goes to so and so, that bookcase (is for you)'.
INTERVIEWER: Would you not do that because you think that the children would sort it out between themselves?
MAVIS: I think they would do yes. Because they're good. They're great friends. I don't think they would fall out.
(Mavis Douglas, 50s, second marriage, home owner)

Although the drama of a will – especially if its contents are unknown – dominates the popular imagery associated with inheritance, in many cases the reality of passing on property is much more banal or (in the case of personal items) more private and individual.

Divisions of property

The point at which property is passed on from one person to others is also the point at which kinship becomes visible, and indeed constituted, in a distinctive way. Focusing on this point enables us to see clearly how people conceptualise the shape of their families, the relative claims of different individuals upon them, and the way in which material property is used to express these relationships. For the most part, these issues are taken for granted and submerged in daily life. They come to the surface and are available for inspection, as it were, when a person is writing a will or expressing an informal view about what should happen to their property, or following a death, when we see relatives responding with approval or concern to the way in which property has actually been transmitted.

We shall therefore explore data about divisions of property from our three studies, looking at both *what patterns are preferred* and *the meanings associated with the patterns*. Our three studies give us access to different types of data on this topic:

- The wills study provides data on patterns of bequeathing through the mechanism of a will. It enables us to map preferred patterns for a representative sample of testators and thus gives a broad picture of how people who write wills conceptualise their own kin group for the purposes of inheritance. However, it must be remembered that only a minority of the population does write a will; the property of the rest would be disposed of according to intestacy law. For this group, we know *who* gets their property. We can make some deductions about the underlying concepts of kinship that this demonstrates, but the evidence here is only indirect.

- The solicitors study provides data from a non-representative (although quite diverse) group of solicitors about their role in helping clients to determine the disposition of their property. This enables us to see whether the solicitors themselves are operating with concepts of family and kinship as they relate to the disposition of property, and whether these concepts are congruent with those of their clients.
- The interview study provides data about the way in which individuals handle inheritance issues in their own families, in some cases including several members of the same family whose accounts can be compared. As far as data on the division of property are concerned, they can be used to examine people's own experiences of past inheritance, their own future intentions, and the underlying models of family and kinship that they utilise when talking about the ownership and transmission of property.

Who gives what to whom?

We begin by using our various data sets to build up a picture of how property is disposed of in practice. We have already noted that English law gives a notable degree of freedom to each individual to decide what should happen to his or her property after death. In principle, this could produce a distribution that is entirely random. In practice it does not. Clear patterns of distribution are visible in our wills data and are broadly confirmed from our other data sets. It is therefore possible to consider what patterns of distribution can tell us about people's concepts of kinship.

A family matter

Data from our wills study show that *the kin group is dominant* when people make bequests. In our wills sample, 92 per cent of testators named at least one relative as a beneficiary, whereas only

17 per cent named a non-relative (such as a friend or neighbour) and only 9 per cent named an organisation (such as a church or charity).

So inheritance is very much a 'family matter' in the sense that property passes very largely, although not exclusively, to kin. When people make positive choices about the disposition of their property they do think first of their kin group. The same pattern is reflected in our interviews with solicitors, whose discussion of their approach to advising clients is dominated by the claims of kin, principally spouses, children and grandchildren. This is not surprising, given that a key consideration for solicitors when giving professional advice is how to avoid claims under family provision legislation against the will that has been written (Finch *et al.* 1996). Such claims could be made only by kin, except where another person could demonstrate economic dependence on the deceased. However, it is also evident that the solicitors whom we interviewed themselves viewed families as having the first claim. As one said to us, he always tried to follow the client's wishes but did have his own views: 'Families should come first, before the dogs' home – even though I am a passionate supporter of dogs.'

Which kin are the main beneficiaries? Under intestacy legislation, the main beneficiaries would be a surviving spouse plus children, in specified proportions depending on the size of the estate. In addition to providing for a surviving spouse, intestacy rules focus upon the blood line and favour descendant relatives over ascendant, close kin over more distant (see Finch *et al.* 1996, chapter 2, for further discussion).

Where the deceased has written a will, our evidence shows a similar pattern, although with more subtleties. It is helpful at this stage to distinguish between two different types of will, which we call 'total estate' and 'composite'. A total estate will is one where property is not differentiated. The testator writes a will that simply rolls up all his or her possessions into a single package and then bequeaths this in specified proportions to named individuals. Sometimes it all goes to a single individual. A composite will is one where different items are specified in the will and bequeathed to named individuals. Typically this might include specified sums of money to each grandchild, named items of jewellery or household objects to named individuals, a house and its contents to the spouse. Such wills – if they have been correctly drawn up – will then roll the rest of the testator's possessions (the 'residue') into a single package and bequeath that in specified proportions. The residue may sometimes consist of the major part of the assets of the estate, and therefore sometimes the value of the residue is quite close to the value of the total estate. However, it is not the value of estates that concerns us so much as the way in which people think about dividing them. From this perspective, all composite wills are different from total estate wills in that they introduce an element of *individuality of gift*, which is absent from a total estate will.

In the sections following, we draw on the distinction between total estate and composite wills to delineate patterns of transmission to different kin.

A surviving spouse

Our wills sample is split almost equally between total estate wills (52 per cent) and composite wills (48 per cent), indicating that roughly half the population of will makers includes an element of individuality of gift. However, the distinction between these two groups is not solely a matter of personal preference. There is an element of predictability about this, related to the marital status of the will maker, because 25 per cent of all our wills are total estate wills bequeathing everything to a surviving spouse, whereas only 12 per cent of composite wills include a spouse. Conversely, 36 per cent of our wills are composite wills in which a spouse is not mentioned (and we have made the assumption that this means that there is no surviving spouse).

It is clear therefore that the form that wills take, and the provisions contained therein, are strongly influenced by whether the testator has a surviving spouse at the time of writing the will. Where a testator was married at the time of writing a will, the process seems to be, for many people, a simple legal mechanism for transferring all assets between spouses. Where there is no surviving spouse, it would appear that many people start to think in a different way about the disposition of their possessions, and the patterns that they produce can be quite complex. We can see this by looking at the most complex of our wills: those with many testators named, with complex divisions of property or with substitutes provided in case the first choice of beneficiary dies before the testator. These wills tend to be written by people who are not married (or do not have a surviving spouse) at the time of writing the will, by women, by older people and by people whose estates are of relatively high value. But within those tendencies there are considerable patterns of variation (for more details see Finch et al. 1996).

Gender is a significant dimension here. Men are more likely than women to write total estate wills with spouse as beneficiary. Women are more likely than men to write some form of complex will. While there may be an interesting range of explanations for this, it is not surprising on purely demographic grounds. Given differences in male and female life expectancy, and the tendency for husbands to be older than their wives, women are more likely to be the survivors of the couple. In situations where assets pass 'automatically' to the survivor, this means that some women may effectively 'control' inheritance to descendant generations (Finch and Hayes 1995). We shall return to this issue in our discussion of gender in Chapter 7.

The dominance of the claims of spouses is also supported by our interview data, although in a rather curious way. In essence, people do not mention inheritance from their own spouse (if they are widowed). Nor do they mention bequeathing to spouses (if they are married) when talking about their intentions for their own property. Just over two-thirds of our interview sample of eighty-four told us that they have inherited something in the past, although for the majority this was a small item of personal property or a cash sum. Twenty interviewees reported that they had inherited something major (a share of, or all of, a house or testator's estate), most of them in older age groups. However, only one person includes bequests from a spouse as part of her account of past experiences of inheritance. If one examines the interview transcripts of other widows and widowers, they are simply silent on this issue. They may mention inheriting from parents or parents-in-law, or even other kin, but not their deceased spouse. A similar pattern occurred when we asked our interviewees about their own bequeathing intentions. Only seven mentioned bequests to a spouse, two of whom said that they would bequeath to their spouse exclusively. The much more dominant theme was bequests to descendant generations: children, grandchildren, nieces and nephews.

We draw from this the rather significant conclusion that *people do not think that property passing to a spouse constitutes inheritance.* Passing on one's property is thought of as predominantly transmission to the next generation. This is what people think of when 'inheritance' is mentioned. This holds despite the fact that most property does in fact pass to the spouse if there is a survivor. This is true whether the transmission takes place through a will, through intestacy laws or through the transfer of property as part of the administration of the estate, which would include property held jointly by spouses. Estimates of property transfers based on Inland Revenue statistics indicate this, although it is very difficult to estimate the extent of transmission to spouses since many house properties are jointly owned (Hamnett 1996).

We therefore further deduce that the transmission of property to a surviving spouse is seen as a separate and distinct process with its own underlying logic. Although in legal terms transmission to a spouse constitutes inheritance no more and no less than to a son or daughter, in English culture these are two distinct processes. The basis of this difference is the (for the most part unquestioned) assumption that married individuals hold property in common. This is an assumption that has replaced the earlier custom that married men were the holders of property. Indeed, winning the rights of married women to hold property was one of the early victories for the women's movement in this country. However, it is only in the second half of the twentieth century that we have seen the growth of joint property holding as the norm, alongside the spread of home ownership, which raises this issue in a form with particular resonance for inheritance.

What our inheritance data underline is just how widespread and how strong is the assumption that spouses have an automatic right to each other's property, especially to house property and personal effects. This general and strong expectation clearly underscores the patterns in the complex families we discussed in Chapter 2, where a second spouse is expected to inherit everything for use during his or her lifetime, irrespective of the existence of step-children. Transmission to a surviving spouse is so much taken for granted that most of our interviewees do not think to mention it and do not count it as inheritance. This is irrespective of the actual legal status of ownership and of whether the transmission has taken place through administrative transfer of assets, through a will or through intestacy law.

The following excerpt from our interview data illustrates these points about the distinctive nature of transfers to a surviving spouse. It is from Sandra Fisher, who is talking about inheritance from her parents, who in their later years owned and ran a guest house in Blackpool:

INTERVIEWER: Do you know if your father left a will?
SANDRA: I don't think he did, because I don't really think that he had anything at that point apart from the house. My mother may even have had that in her name – the guest house that they had bought. We were hard up at that point and I don't think that there was anything for him to leave.
INTERVIEWER: And you think that the guest house was in your mother's name?
SANDRA: It might have been. Or even if it was in joint names it would have gone to her automatically, wouldn't it?
(Sandra Fisher, 40s, married, home owner)

The logic of Sandra's answer about her parents' property is that the house – their main asset and also their business in this particular case – was not available for transmission to anyone other than her mother at the time of her father's death. She does not know the structure of ownership between her parents, but that is of no consequence: her mother would take possession of this asset in any event. It was therefore not relevant for her father to write a will, since he had – as she defines it – nothing to be passed on. This same logic is followed by more or less all our interviewees, with the frequent observation that an individual has 'just a house' to pass on. If there is a surviving spouse, this is taken to mean that there is no disposable estate, since she or he will simply take full possession of it.

Thus although English law accords testamentary freedom to all of us, most people do not regard that as relevant if they have a spouse who will survive them. It is particularly noteworthy that children do not see themselves as having claims on the major asset of a deceased parent if the other parent is still alive. This contrasts sharply with jurisdictions operating under the civil code, where it is children who inherit even if one of their parents is still living.

Patterns of bequests to kin

We have already noted that beneficiaries are predominantly members of the testator's kin network. Apart from spouses, who gets included and what do they receive? Our data from the wills sample enable us to track the answers to these questions quite precisely, and we have discussed this matter in detail in Finch *et al.* (1996). We shall provide only a brief summary here.

All discussions of this topic must begin with the warning that there is considerable variation in the way property is disposed of. Aside from the special position of the surviving spouse, people do appear to make quite individual decisions about who gets what. There are differences in the form of property disposal (by total estate or by composite will), in the type of individual items that are named in wills, and in the range of kin who are included. In that sense, the population of will makers takes full advantage of the freedom that English law affords.

That said, there are discernible patterns. In general, the identity of people included as beneficiaries, and what each person receives, is related to three separate but interwoven factors: genealogical closeness to the testator, generational position and whether a person can be seen as 'next of kin'. The closer a person is in genealogical terms, the more likely she or he is to receive a major gift. (In this discussion, we are using the term 'major gift' to refer to a significant portion of the testator's estate.) That could be a share of the total estate, or the residue once personal gifts have been extracted, or specifically a house. We make no assumption about monetary value when we use the term 'major gift'. The value of estates varies greatly. The point is that, from the testator's perspective, however much he or she has to bequeath, a gift of the total estate or residue represents a major slice of the assets that are being passed on.

We begin with the different ways in which children and grandchildren are treated. In our wills sample, 36 per cent contain gifts to children but only 12 per cent to grandchildren, who are one step more distant. Although some of this difference may be accounted for by age (some of our testators may not have had grandchildren at the time when they were writing their will), there is a also a clear contrast in the type of gift received. The most common gift to a child is a 'major' gift, although the likelihood of receiving this depends on whether there is a surviving spouse. Taking only those wills that mention children as beneficiaries but where there is no mention of a spouse, children are extremely likely to receive a major gift – 97 per cent of wills of this nature leave children a share of either the total estate or the residue. However, in wills where there is a surviving spouse as well as children, this figure drops to 34 per cent. By contrast, the typical gift to grandchildren is a small cash sum, received by 66 per cent of grandchildren in our sample; only 16 per cent receive a share of the total estate or residue.

In generational terms, there is a preference for looking 'down' the generations. Spouses apart, only 18 per cent of wills contain bequests to someone in the same generation – all to siblings. This can be compared with 17 per cent, about the same number, that contain bequests to a niece or nephew – a position that is genealogically more distant but is in a descendant generation. Thus the factor of genealogy and generation appear to operate separately from each other. Added to them is the 'next-of-kin' factor. Although this is more difficult to discern from wills (especially since wills provide no information about kin who may exist but who receive no gift), we deduce that there is a tendency to identify a person or persons who are closest to the testator in genealogical terms, and to single them out for the biggest gifts. This is clearly true when there is a surviving spouse, as we have already indicated. If there is no surviving spouse, it seems that children are substitute recipients, in a sense, of the major share. The same applies where neither spouse nor children are named in the will. Where the genealogically closest people mentioned are nieces and nephews, in 42 per cent of cases they receive a share of the total estate or residue – a situation that contrasts with the typical gift in other wills, which would be a cash sum. However, this figure of 42 per cent is lower than the proportion of children who receive a major gift where they are in the next-of-kin position (97 per cent), indicating that the next-of-kin factor does appear but does not totally overrule genealogy and generation.

Turning to our data from interviews, the patterns reported match quite closely the data from wills. We asked our interviewees whether they had ever inherited from someone else and they reported a total of 102 examples (some people had inherited more than once). Forty-five of these examples were gifts from one or both parents. The next most common was inheritance from a grandparent (seventeen) or an aunt/uncle (eighteen). When we asked them whether they might inherit something in the future, parents were much the most commonly mentioned source.

We also asked our interviewees about their own bequeathing intentions and whether they had already written a will. A total of

44 per cent of interviewees reported that they have written a will, with women a little more likely than men to have done this, and people over sixty much more likely to have written a will than younger people. At the other end of the spectrum, almost a quarter of our interviewees had given so little thought to passing on their own property that we have no meaningful data about their bequeathing intentions. About two-thirds of our interviewees (fifty-six people) say that they will bequeath some or all of their assets to children, with other kin being mentioned much less frequently (for example, only eleven people mention grandchildren and eight mention nieces and nephews).

The type of gift mentioned in relation to our interviewees' own bequeathing intentions also reflects the wills data. Bequests to spouses and children centre on the total estate (with sometimes the house being singled out for special mention). Where other kin are mentioned, the focus shifts to cash gifts or to items of personal property. Thus for the most part people's thoughts about the disposition of their own property are fairly instrumental and practical, focused upon arrangements for passing on their major assets.

When talking about gifts that they themselves have received in the past, interviewees are much more likely to mention items of personal property. In total, our interviewees reported sixty-four examples of having inherited personal items. Exactly half of these examples were bequests from parents to children, and the rest were very varied in their source. In the great majority of cases, the item inherited was a piece of jewellery (including watches), with a tendency – although not an absolute rule – for gifts to pass down the gender-specific line of descent, from father to son or mother to daughter. These data suggest that bequeathing personal items is actually much more extensive than is reflected in our wills data, probably because these items may be passed on 'informally' outside the will. What our interview data capture – by contrast with the wills data – are bequests that people have vested with enough significance to remember and report. It would appear that this produces a rather different pattern from formal bequeathing, with gifts of personal property thus 'remembered' more frequently than their appearance in wills would suggest. We return to this issue in detail in Chapter 6.

In part this is explained by the apparent preference of solicitors for keeping items of personal property out of wills. Although most of those we interviewed said that they have to follow the wishes of the client, and do indeed ask whether clients wish to make any bequests of personal effects, in reality they will discourage long lists of such items. As one put it, if faced with a long list of specific bequests she would encourage the client to 'tighten up a bit', suggesting that they give their executors a list of such items outside the will.

Principles of dividing property

So far we have discussed who gets included as a beneficiary and what different types of beneficiary typically receive. Given that position in the kin network is by far the most significant factor in both of these, it is relevant to ask how gifts are actually divided. We have, for example, shown that typically (if there is no surviving spouse) children would get a share of the total estate or residue, grandchildren would get a cash gift, and so on. But does each child receive the same proportionate share? Does each grandchild receive the same amount of cash? In other words, is genealogical position as such the key factor, or do testators think more about the *individuals* to whom they are bequeathing and leave one child a larger share than another, give one grandchild a larger sum than the rest?

Our wills data suggest that the most prominent principle of division is to give equal shares or gifts to people who occupy the same genealogical position relative to the testator; however, while this is certainly the dominant principle it is not completely invariable (see Finch *et al.* 1996: chapter 5). In total, 22 per cent of our wills sample contain examples of differential treatment (people of the same kin type receiving gifts that are not the same). However, the majority of these cases cover bequests of items of personal property where, for example, one sibling receives an item of jewellery while another receives a piece of furniture. It may well be that, within the family, it is understood that these gifts are actually of roughly equivalent value, although we cannot tell that from the wills. It is much more rare for wills to contain bequests that are clearly unequal, for example in the sense of leaving different proportions of the residue to different children. Only 5 per cent of our wills had differential provisions of this kind. In addition, 3 per cent of wills contain another sort of differential treatment where people of the same kin type are accorded different beneficiary status. This means that, for example, one niece inherits directly as a first-choice beneficiary while another will inherit only as a substitute beneficiary – that is, where the person first named in the will has already died before the testator dies.

The general pattern in wills is therefore that differential treatment of a kind that clearly treats similar beneficiaries unequally is rare, although it can be found. It is very unlikely to occur with relationships of direct descent (children and grandchildren). Where it does occur, it is likely to involve nieces, nephews or cousins. In these relationships, it would appear that people do not feel they need to treat every cousin or nephew on equal terms. However, for children and grandchildren it would seem that the impulse to equal treatment is much stronger, almost invariable.

This could be explained in several ways. Our solicitors' interviews suggest that it is an automatic assumption by both themselves and their clients that children will be treated equally, although under English law this is not required. Many solicitors interviewed said that clients had only a hazy view of what they really wanted when they first sought professional advice and, as a result, most get a fairly standard package. There was very little, if any, experience of clients wanting to use a will to cut out a particular child or grandchild, for example. This argument suggests that equal treatment of children is seen as the norm and tends to be followed unless there is a strong reason to do otherwise. That would fit with a second type of explanation, namely that equal treatment of children in wills is entirely consistent with evidence about how family life operates in general. Our analysis of inheritance in families with experience of divorce, separation, repartnering and step-relationships (see Chapter 2) indicates that step-children may also be included in this 'equal treatment' regime.

In the interview data, it is very clear that the principle of equal treatment of children reigns supreme when it comes to the division of major assets. Often the principle is implicit in what interviewees say, which is an indication that it is really taken for granted rather than a matter upon which each individual might take her or his own decision. The principle is taken for granted whether an interviewee is talking from the perspective of testator (about how his or her own property might be divided) or as a beneficiary (about what has been received in the past or might be received in the future). The view also seems common to all interviewees of whatever age, gender or material circumstances. The following example is typical. The interviewee is discussing the distribution of money from the estate of an aunt.

> She was intestate, they call it, and the money had to be distributed between all the family. My mum had eight brothers and sisters and we had to find all the relatives, all the children's children and whatever. If they had died their children got a twelfth of a twelfth and so forth.
> (Ted Beech, 70, married, home owner)

In some cases, people are more explicit about the principle of equal division and, where this occurs, the emphasis is usually on the possibilities for conflict if the principle of equal division were to be breached.

> INTERVIEWER: Do you think that inheritance can cause problems?
> JOSIE: Oh yes, I do.
> INTERVIEWER: With or without wills?
> JOSIE: Well I suppose it depends how you leave your will. You know, if you have left it to one child and not to the other two, it would cause eruptions.
> (Josie Lewis, 40s, married, home owner)

Simple though the principle of equal divisions appears, some of our interviewees are conscious of the practical difficulties of accomplishing it. We have already shown the possible complexities in the case of complex families (see Chapter 2), but there are other variations on this theme. For example, Ron Beattie aspires to produce an equitable outcome between his children but sees that this may be difficult to achieve if his son and daughter occupy very different positions in the housing market:

> It's not just a case that they will have equal shares, because that would be unfair. You've got to take into account what circumstances they are in, how they are likely to benefit. Particularly now it comes into the picture more than it did before, this house business, more than it did six years ago because the prices have gone up so. So you've got to give much closer attention to that point – which one is likely to be

in need of it. It's not just a question of splitting it down the middle and dividing it all up.

(Ron Beattie, 70s, married, home owner)

Most people are more concerned with dividing their property using principles of strict equivalence than with whether or not the different life circumstances of their children mean that some will end up with greater material wealth than others. Strict equivalence can be perceived as difficult if the major part of the parent's estate consists of property. The following example comes from Souresh Khan, a doctor of Asian descent with a British-born wife, who owns several different properties:

> Our will says that if something happens to both of us, then the boys get a share equally. But we haven't gone into detail. I think we have been a bit lazy there, actually we should go into more detail. Because we have got some properties which can't be shared half and half. You can't tell whether they are going to get on with each other later in life, and it might not be easy to split it at the time. We have got no fluid money. That's quite easy to distribute because you can do it 50–50. But when it comes to sharing house property, you really have to sell it for the sake of getting the money to share it equally.
>
> (Souresh Khan, 40s, married, home owner)

The principle of equal divisions between children, strong though it is, is not unbreachable according to our interviewees. It would seem that there are circumstances that justify selecting a specific child for special treatment while maintaining the fundamental principle of equality.

These circumstances fall into two categories. First, there are circumstances where one child has a particular economic tie to his or her parents. In these circumstances, it seems to be accepted that this child should benefit more from the parents' estate than do the others. We have six cases of this cited in our interview data, one of which comes from Rosie King, who is talking about the distribution of her parents' estate. This includes a working farm, on which her brother is employed. Rosie regards it as absolutely right that he should inherit a larger share of the farm, but when it comes to their parents' planned retirement home – a property in which he would have no bigger stake than any other sibling – Rosie would expect this to be divided equally.

> My brother has a third share of the farm, which he has worked all his life for. We left home. We've done nothing towards the working of the farm. So my brother is entitled. If my mum and dad retired they would sell their stock. Tom would have a third of it, so he would have a third of everything they owned to start up his own farm. Two-thirds would belong to my mum and dad. They would sell it, and provide themselves with a bungalow. And when that bungalow was sold – after my mum and dad (have died) – all the money that was left would be shared equally between us.
> (Rosie King, 30, married, home owner)

A second type of circumstance that appears to justify special treatment is where there is a clear and distinct need or claim on the part of one child. Fifteen of our interviewees indicated that they either knew of such circumstances or could envisage that special bequests would be appropriate should they arise. The most common examples given were cases where children or young adults have remained resident in the parents' home and in that sense are still dependent on their parents, while others have left to form independent households. A good example comes from our interview with Marianne Horner, who was 21 years old when we interviewed her. Marianne was married with her own household, but one sister still lived in the parental home. As things stand at present, she would expect the distribution of her parents' estate to be unequal to reflect that. However, she would be upset if that continued into a future when her sister had become independent:

> I think if my parents were to write a will now, if they were to die while Jane is still at college, I think she would be left with a larger portion than me or John. Because the two of us, we are independent. We can basically look after ourselves. But if it's in the future, well then I think we would be left with equal parts. I hope we would (laughs).
> (Marianne Horner, 20s, married, home owner)

Although the co-residence of immature children provides the largest and clearest group of comments about treating an individual child as a 'special case', this is not the only circumstance mentioned. The long-term disability of the child is another example given. In a sense this mirrors the argument about immaturity, both types of example being about the specific dependence of children on parents.

The other circumstances that one could envisage as a possible reason for special treatment is where one child has cared for one or both parents in old age. However, only two people mention the special claims of a child based on this circumstance, yet we have many more cases where such caring relationships have existed. These two cases are as follows:

> Everything [of my mother's] was divided. But my sister had looked after my mother mostly when she was ill, because I was working. I had to work to support my daughter. So she got the choice of things. We sort of halved them.
> (Meg Russell, 70s, separated then widowed, home owner)

ELLEN: My mother used to say 'I've left everything to you'. She always said that when I saw her.

INTERVIEWER: How did you feel about her leaving it to you and not your brother?

ELLEN: Well I didn't think my brother deserved it. He used to live a quarter of an hour's walk away. She saw more of me – and I lived two hundred miles away – than she ever did of him.
(Ellen Beech, 60s, married, home owner)

Although looked at from different perspectives – one was herself the main supporter, the other was not – both seem clear that having been the main carer for an ailing parent is justification for special treatment in the distribution of the parent's estate.

These examples indicate that, without violating the general principle of equal treatment, there is room for an element of individuality even in the distribution of major assets to children. This occurs in circumstances where there is a clear economic tie between parents and children. The fact that it applies to only a small number of circumstances reported to us indicates that normally there is no such tie. Where it does occur, the economic link has the effect of modifying the tendency – otherwise universal – to treat all children equally in the distribution of major gifts.

The distribution of items of personal property is different. Differentiation between individuals is much more common. We have already indicated that the people whom we interviewed were much more likely to talk about personal items that they had inherited than about bequests of more major assets. Taking solely the example of bequests from parents to children, forty-one individuals report forty-five examples of receiving inheritance from a parent. In thirty-two of these instances personal property is mentioned, and in twenty-two cases *only* personal property is mentioned. This contrasts with ten instances of inheriting a parent's estate (or a share of it) and six of inheriting a house. The same pattern is repeated for gifts between other categories of kin. But the striking fact is that even in the case of bequests to children, who are the most likely recipients of the residue where there is no surviving spouse, we have many more instances of people remembering and reporting personal gifts, often of small items that probably had little monetary value. The symbolic importance of inherited items is profoundly significant for our understanding of kinship, and we explore this in depth in Chapter 6.

In this discussion of principles of division we have concentrated mainly on children because it is here that the interweaving of equality and individuality comes across most clearly. Both are present in other relationships, but in different ways. For example, the principle of equality applies equally strongly in the case of grandchildren, but the element of individuality is less strong. It is present, however, with some individuals very much treasuring items inherited from a grandparent – often because they are thereby reminded of their own childhood. In the case of more distant kin, and especially of non-kin, equal treatment is not really an issue, but individuality is – the whole point of leaving a gift to a friend or relative is to acknowledge the nature of the friendship.

Conflicts about divisions

Mention of the topic of inheritance seems generally to conjure up images of conflict between relatives about who gets what. Certainly this theme has underscored countless novels and plays. Before leaving the topic of division of assets, we therefore need to give an overview of what our data say about conflict.

The most notable point about our interviews is that we have very few cases where people actually report experience of the kind of wrangles about bequests that are the stuff of literature and popular culture. We do have a few cases where – it is alleged – relatives sneaked in and took what they wanted before anyone else could get there, but our interviewees gave us no examples from their own experience where a will was contested (although one or two comments indicate that a person may have thought about this, then rejected it). The reality for most people would appear to be smoother, and probably more banal.

However, we do have a couple of rather poignant comments of a more general kind, which show an awareness of the possible ways in which a particular instance of inheritance can subsequently sour relationships:

> The members of my family haven't spoken to each other for years. In fact they don't speak to each other until they are ready to die themselves, which is sad. That's what I am talking about. Sadness. It does bring a lot of sadness – and greed. Wills – they're greed.
> (Sean Flynn, 40s, married, home owner)

In this second extract, the interviewee is expressing the view that the content of wills should be talked about openly in families well in advance of a possible death, especially if the division is not going to be equal:

> They should sit down and say, 'Look, you've been lucky in your life, you've been given everything, he's got nothing. We feel that a big chunk of our money should go to him. And I am sure that you will be quite happy with what we leave you'. I think if you are quite open, then they will be quite happy at that stage. Rather than somebody reads the will and it comes out there. I think it's the shock. That is the problem. That can cause the friendship, or the close relationship between brothers and sisters, to go. Money is an evil thing at the end of the day really.
> (Souresh Khan, 40s, married, home owner)

These views that 'wills are greed' and 'money is an evil thing' would perhaps accord with what many people would expect us to find in a study of inheritance and families. In fact, they represent very much a minority experience, at least in that overt form. The avoidance of conflict is sometimes cited as a reason for making a will, or for making specific provisions (as, for example, in some cases above where people are pondering how to ensure that the division between their children is experienced as equitable). But the experience of conflict *per se* is rare.

Where overt conflict has occurred, it seems to be concerned mainly with one of two circumstances. Either someone unexpected or unauthorised takes away specific personal possessions or, if it concerns major assets, the story usually concerns a more distant relative who gets hold of a share when they have no real moral claim. It seems as if the involvement of wider kin creates more opportunities for judgements about moral entitlement to come into play, and at this point people bring into the frame their views about the past and present behaviour of their kin, quite outside the question of inheritance.

It is in data on these cases where we meet characters who take on the role of the villain of the piece – or, at the very least, characters who are undeserving of their good fortune. The villains are always beneficiaries. Testators are never cast in the role of villain. There seems to be an absolute bar on treating a testator's intentions as inappropriate or unworthy. The following provide illustrations. In the first extract, the situation relates to the ownership of Jill Pettifer's grandmother's house and a dispute with her mother's brother. Jill's family actually lived in the house with the grandmother; the uncle did not. Jill's own mother died before her grandmother.

> My grandmother hadn't written a will because she was suffering from senile dementia. She got too difficult to handle and she ended up in residential care. Then my mother died. Then my mother's brother decided that half the property should be his. It caused quite a stir. It meant my dad having to sell, and there was still my younger sister at home at the time. My uncle insisted that my dad sold the house and gave him his half share. It was quite traumatic for my dad. It caused quite a rift because this uncle didn't need the money. It went through court and everything. It was all done legally. It was quite upsetting.
>
> (Jill Pettifer, 40s, divorced, home owner)

In the second extract, Rachael Harvey is anticipating a situation that she wants to take action to avoid:

> I said that I didn't want any of my husband's family to have anything. That's why we made a will that, if anything happened to us, it goes to the godchildren. I mean there's certain members of my husband's family who I wouldn't want to have any of my hard-earned cash.
> (Rachel Harvey, 40s, married, home owner)

The 'villains' in these two examples are in-laws and an uncle. Other common candidates for this role are step-relatives, as we showed in Chapter 2. The legal claims of such relatives are not really the issue, as Jill Pettifer's quote above shows clearly. Even if a relative in this category has the legal right to inherit, their past behaviour may lead others to reject their claim on moral grounds, even though they know that this can have no practical effect.

However, we must emphasise that these colourful and intriguing conflicts around inheritance represent a very minor theme in the practical experience of our interviewees. For the most part, they are no more than cautionary tales whose real value is to expose cultural assumptions rather than indicators of lived reality.

Conclusion

The data reviewed in this chapter suggest that people treat the division of the major parts of their estate as a relatively straightforward matter, certainly if they have children. Despite the freedom of testamentary disposition that English law allows, most people do not give a great deal of detailed thought to what should happen to their main assets. These generally go to the children and get divided equally, and this outcome is more or less taken for granted. Only if there are no children is the choice treated as more open. The principle of equal division can and should be breached if there is a specific reason for doing so and, specifically, where there is an economic tie between parent and one child. But in the absence of such reasons, equal division is assumed. For most people, the experience of inheritance, certainly of major assets, is thus straightforward and is not accompanied by the kind of colourful disputes that are the stuff of popular imagination about inheritance.

The act of bequeathing, as far as these major assets is concerned, is not notably linked to personal attachment or the individuality of relationships in most cases, especially where there are surviving children. That is not to say that the act of bequeathing to children is purely mechanical, divorced from family attachments, but at most the expression of attachment is indirect – the symbol of a lifetime's commitment as a parent – rather than a specific gift from one individual to another. The individual gift, specially selected to pass from one person to another and to symbolise their relationship, comes through bequests of personal items. This practice is widespread, and much of it probably occurs informally, outside a will. A wide range of people are, as it were, eligible to receive such gifts, although not all testators use that freedom or want to. Children often receive personal gifts even if they are also getting major assets.

The model of family and kinship that emerges from these data contains features that are both fixed and fluid. The fixed points are the absolute priority accorded to a surviving spouse, to the extent that no one else expects to inherit in these circumstances. The position of children is also relatively fixed in that patterns of bequest are quite predictable. Beyond the spouse, descendant generations take priority, but this really means children as far as major gifts are concerned. Thus on one level the image of kinship emerging from these data is restricted to spouse plus children. In so far as inheritance is used to mark out the boundaries of significant family relationships, the dominant model is very confined. However, this leaves out of account the bequest of gifts of personal property and small cash sums, whose monetary value may be insignificant but which, as we have indicated, seem to figure more in people's lived experience of inheritance than a simple analysis of major gifts would suggest. If one takes these into account, then grandchildren and nieces and nephews may come into the frame. This therefore introduces the fluid element into the picture. Individuals can and do use inheritance to mark the boundaries of *their own* kin group.

This pattern is broadly consistent with an individualistic kinship structure, which we discussed in Chapter 1. The individual is clearly at the centre of his or her own network. Parent–child relations hold a central place. No discernible distinction is made between women and men as beneficiaries when property is being divided, although we have noted that, as the likely survivors of 'the couple', women as testators are more likely to 'control' the inheritance of property down the generations. However, these bequeathing patterns, which display individualistic concepts of kinship, come into play only where there is no surviving spouse. Where there is, she or he has an overriding claim.

The data reviewed in this chapter also offer some interesting insights into concepts of property, in particular whether there is a common stake across generations. We have seen that there are circumstances in which a common stake clearly exists, in the sense that there is an economic tie between a parent and a particular child: a disabled child with a long-term dependency on parents; a son who has become a partner in a family farming enterprise; a daughter who has become the main carer for an elderly parent. In these circumstances, our interviewees accept that it may be right for this economic tie to be acknowledged through inheritance. However, this happens rarely. In most families there is no economic tie between parents and their adult children, and parental property is divided through inheritance on a strict basis of equal shares.

Our data reviewed so far seem to confirm that there is no common stake in property in most families, but also that this can be modified in particular circumstances. In the following chapter, we continue to explore whether and how a sense of 'family property' comes into play in the context of English kinship, and we shift the focus from transmission to questions about receiving and using inherited property.

Chapter 4
Moral dilemmas

Introduction

Up to now our focus has been upon *transmission* of property. But who gives what to whom, and how it is divided, are only parts of the picture in which we are interested. In this chapter, we want to shift the focus away from transmission and on to what is involved in *receiving* an inheritance. For present purposes, we shall confine our discussion to the inheritance of money and major assets, although we shall return to a consideration of personal possessions in Chapter 6. Specifically, in this chapter we are interested in what beneficiaries do with money they inherit, how those decisions get made, what meaning they have, and what that tells us about kinship. Our data suggest that the inheritance of money poses particular moral dilemmas for beneficiaries.

Receiving an inheritance is a distinctive experience, set apart from the more routine or ceremonial practices of gift exchange in families. We know from anthropological and sociological studies since Mauss' classic *The Gift* that gift exchange is an important medium for the shaping of kin relationships, and that the ritual elements and the demeanour of the participants in the process are central (Berking 1999; Cheal 1988; Goffman 1972; Mauss 1954). Berking argues that 'The material offering, the ceremonial handing over, the proofs of thankfulness – these frame an exchange in which a great deal is always at stake' (1999: 3). However, inheritance poses problems in this respect. Usually there is no process of handing over, ceremonial or otherwise, directly from donor to recipient. Similarly, 'proofs of thankfulness' cannot be achieved directly between beneficiary and testator. In the absence of clear rules of etiquette, and also of a living donor to whom a recipient can express gratitude, people struggle to work out the proper thing to do. Our data suggest that inheriting money or assets prompts people to make *active moral* decisions, and that these are central to our understanding of kinship.

In focusing on active moral decisions, we are situating ourselves within a growing body of research and theory that argues at least two things: first, that 'ordinary people' see morality as central to their lives, in the sense that people are concerned with the morality of their actions (and, we would argue, their thoughts); and, second, that the morality of people's actions – or people's moral actions – is not derived from abstract ethical principles that are either generally agreed upon or imposed by 'ethical experts', but have to be worked out in concrete situations and, we would argue, most crucially in relationships with others (Bauman 1992; Benhabib 1992; Finch and Mason 1993; Hekmann 1995; Mason 1996a; Sevenhuijsen 1998; Smart and Neale 1999). These perspectives are relevant to our discussion of inheritance in various ways. Inheritance is of course about material resources, yet the passing on and receiving of money via inheritance is about much more than material transactions, as is clear from our discussion so far. In this chapter, we examine these issues specifically.

Inheriting money

We are including a range of types of inherited gift within the term 'inheriting money'. First, there are specified cash sums. Twenty-two of our interviewees report having themselves received this kind of bequest in the past. Second, there are bequests of someone's 'estate', or a share of it. These kinds of bequest invariably include money and often houses, which are almost always sold by beneficiaries and hence converted into money (Finch and Hayes 1994). As we shall show in Chapter 5, our data suggest that houses that form part of a total estate are treated as assets for disposal in this way by both testators and beneficiaries: it is intended that the value of the house be transmitted rather than that the house itself be preserved. Twenty-five of our respondents report having received someone's 'estate' or a share of it, or a share of a house or land. As well as these examples of direct experience of inheriting money, estates and houses, many more people gave us third party examples of these kinds of inheritance, and we have included third party examples where they are relevant in our discussion here. And many people who inherit money also receive bequests of personal property and keepsakes, the transmission of which we discuss later.

Our discussion of the use of inherited money draws on our interview data alone, since our wills and solicitors data sets cannot tell us about these aspects of inheritance. We are focusing on a stage when all issues surrounding the transmission of resources have been settled. At this stage, the beneficiary is on her or his own, freed from legal constraints except for those relatively rare cases where the will has established a trust, which then restricts the use of funds (Finch *et al.* 1996).

There is a range of ways in which people in our study report using, spending and disposing of inherited money, and many people use a cash bequest or a share of an estate in more than one way. Here is an example from Helena Muhkerjee, who is talking about what she did with a large bequest of money from an aunt:

> We put some of it into his [husband's] business ... Some of it I invested, and then when we bought this house I took out the investment and put the money into a contribution towards this property. We put some money in a special account to pay for our daughter's education because she goes to a private school. And I mean yes we could do a few frivolous things. I bought myself a few nice things to wear and we had a lovely holiday. But we didn't go bananas because, you know, we did put some in the business and we were sensible about it, what we did with it. And as I said I mean you know, there's very little to see in pounds, shillings and pence for it now, but it's locked up in other ways. I mean, it's in bricks and mortar, in here.
> (Helena Muhkerjee, 40s, married, home owner)

Helena's example of using money in a range of ways is fairly typical, although the size of her gift enabled more flexibility than for many of our beneficiaries, who might simply have inherited a few hundred pounds. Our data tell us quite a lot about these processes, although we should note that we did not attempt an analysis of expenditure patterns, nor did we ask people to itemise every single way in which they used inherited money, or to try to quantify how much they spent on what. Such data might have been difficult to elicit, however, since it is significant that when we asked about what they themselves had inherited and what they did with it, people were much less forthcoming about money than about specific items of personal property like jewellery, watches or china tea services. However, the fact remains that many people do inherit money and have to make decisions about what to do with it.

On the face of it, there are three broad options: give some or all of the money away, keep or invest it, or spend it. We shall discuss each of these in turn, although it is important to note that the boundaries between them are not entirely clear-cut. For example, money can be spent on other people; money can be spent on something that is perceived to be an investment, such as a house; money can be placed in an investment account, not so much as an investment *per se* but in order to postpone having to make decisions about what to do with it; and money can be used in a combination of ways, as in the example of Helena Muhkerjee above.

Giving inherited money away

We have sixteen reports in our data of people giving inherited money (some or all of it) away, including some third party examples. The majority of our interviewees, therefore, did not report giving inherited money away. Our examples are split almost equally three ways between those where people passed money down a generation, to their own children; those who passed money or land across their own generation to siblings; and those who passed money up a generation, in every case to a widowed mother. We can find no examples in our data of people giving inherited money to more genealogically distant kin, or to individuals who were not kin, or to other bodies or charities. There is a rough gender balance in people giving money away, although the numbers are small. Slightly more women than men overall do this, except in the category of 'passing up' a generation to a mother, where more men than women are involved. Five out of seven of the 'passing across' examples come from people of Asian origin (who were a minority in our sample as a whole). Three of these involve people who had inherited, along with their siblings, an equal share in land in India, and had passed their share over to brothers still living in India and working the land. Some examples involve inheritance via a will, and some do not. Overall, the examples of giving money away all involve money or land inherited as part or all of an estate rather than as a specified cash gift. This is a significant point, to which we shall return.

These cases are interesting because in some senses they involve beneficiaries apparently acting at odds either with the wishes of a testator as expressed in a will or, where a will has not been made, with the assumptions underpinning administration of estates and intestacy provisions. It is likely that the former is more morally problematic than the latter, because a will contains a formal expression of the deceased person's wishes, so doing something different could be construed (by the actors themselves as well as observers) as 'going against' those wishes. Diverging from legal prescriptions does not carry the same sense of departure from anyone's personal wishes, although it might raise moral problems of a different order.

There seem to be a number of ways of understanding what is happening here, which apply differentially in relation to passing down, passing across and passing up. The first possible explanation is that redistribution of inherited resources is really what the testator wanted and that the participants are merely acting on his or her wishes. Certainly, there is some suggestion that, where people make simple wills (for example, all to a spouse, or all to children), in reality they may expect something to be passed on to children or grandchildren. However, after someone has died it is difficult to determine whether any redistribution is precisely in line with the testator's wishes. It may have more to do with the recipient's own sets of relationships and responsibilities to their own children and grandchildren. Logically, the idea that giving away some inherited money was 'really' what the testator expected fits best with passing down the generations. However, the only example we have of someone telling us that they are directly following the verbal instructions of a testator in redistributing money is one of the 'passing across' cases – Annie Palfrey. Annie is the sole beneficiary of her mother's will:

> My mother left a will, but it was because of my brother being in a religious order, she didn't want the religious order to get the money. Not that she had a great deal, but what she had, she left with me. But with very strict instructions, mind you, verbal instructions, that I was to make sure that he was, always to make sure that he was all right.
> (Annie Palfrey, late 50s, single, private rented accommodation)

The second possible explanation is that one beneficiary (actual or potential) is perceived by others as being particularly deserving, or to have had a pre-existing economic or supportive relationship with the person who has died. As we noted in Chapter 3, this can be a reason for testators to take the unusual step of making substantially unequal bequests to their own children. We argued there that where testators do this, the intention is to produce equality of *outcome* between their children or to acknowledge a specific economic tie. Nonetheless, it is capable of misinterpretation, apparently putting one child in a privileged position. A further complication is that circumstances may have changed since the will was written, making what a testator apparently intended to be a fair or equal distribution look unfair in the light of subsequent events. Alternatively, the family's circumstances may be too complex to cater for in either a will or intestacy provisions.

Notwithstanding these potential hazards, this explanation, that one of the testator's children is perceived by others as particularly deserving, works for all but one (Annie Palfrey) of our 'passing across' cases, five of which involve interviewees of Asian origin. Three of these involve land in India being passed over to brothers remaining in India who are working the land, and they need to be understood in the specific contexts of migration, transnationality of kinship, and the regulation of the transmission and ownership of property in India. Here is an example from Rakesh Singh, whose father had not made a will:

> It usually goes to all the children, wife and all the children, so after his death we went to the court and we all decided it would go to our youngest brother, my mother and my youngest brother [because] you know, my youngest brother, he suffers from polio. We thought in case he doesn't get a job, in case he doesn't get married, put everything as one. He has got married, and got a wife, he's got a son. But that time we just felt, felt in case he can't you know, afford to buy a house, whereas the rest of us we could. So that was the reason. He's in a very good job now.
> (Rakesh Singh, 40s, married, home owner)

These cases, where participants are essentially turning what would have been an equal distribution of money (or land) into unequal shares, are significant in that they breach the principle that children receive equal shares. It may well be that parents would be perfectly happy for children *themselves* to produce an unequal division but do not feel comfortable with the idea of distributing unequally by their own hand.

The third possible explanation for redistribution after an inheritance has been received is that someone is perceived as having been by-passed in the division of an estate, possibly because of unforeseen circumstances (such as a spouse unexpectedly surviving longer than the testator), or perhaps unjustly. This is the best explanation for our 'passing up' cases, all but one of which involve beneficiaries passing money received direct from their fathers in a will 'back' to their widowed mothers. Three of these cases contain hints that the 'by-passing' of a spouse has been perceived as unjust. Here is Betty Hill's account of her husband's actions on receiving a bequest from his father that apparently 'by-passed' his mother:

> He [husband] got very upset because when his father died, he was left everything, but his mother was still alive. His father had left a will that my husband, the eldest boy, had to have everything. His wife wasn't to have anything. Well what happened is that – my husband didn't know anything then – but he got very upset, and he had everything signed over to his mother. He thought well 'I'll do that', and within a matter of a few months she'd married this other man, which my husband didn't know anything about ... and consequently everything went over to her side and my children didn't get anything.
> (Betty Hill, late 50s, widowed, council rented accommodation)

In general, our data suggest that giving inherited money away is not a very common activity, and it can be morally difficult. In our examples, it is done only within a genealogically tight range of kin – parents, children and siblings – and in rather specific circumstances. Significantly, none of the examples involve money inherited as a specified cash amount (as in 'I leave £100 to Susan Smith'). All of our interviewees who gave away inherited money had received it either as a part or total share of an estate in a will where they and other beneficiaries had been named, but as recipients of a proportion of the whole, rather than a specified sum, or via intestacy provision or administration in the absence of a will. None of them appears to have given money away lightly and, significantly, they could all account for their actions, often appearing to have negotiated them with other participants.

There is also evidence of moral hazard in giving money away and 'going against the wishes of the testator', especially if these have been formulated very precisely and 'publicly' in a will. Betty Hill's story, with its implied question 'did his father know something?' has a moral attached, which goes something like 'woe betide anyone who goes against the wishes of the deceased, however just their actions may appear to be'. While this 'moral of the story' does not directly apply to all the cases, giving inherited money away is not a morally safe or easy option – ironically, perhaps, given the sense of moral propriety that we see attached to acts of 'generosity' in kin relationships more generally (Finch and Mason 1993). It appears that people may have to tread a delicate path between 'going against the wishes' of the testator, and showing themselves – if not to be generous – then at least not to be avaricious, as they might by keeping what they and others feel to be more than their fair share.

Keeping and investing money

Keeping inherited money may seem easier than giving it away, although doing one does not, of course, preclude the other. A powerful incentive to keep inherited money may be that it requires less decision making than other courses of action at what may be a difficult time for a beneficiary. People who subsequently give away some inherited money may have kept it for a time while they decided what to do, and people may give some away and keep the rest. Indeed, we have some evidence that giving some away (being 'generous') might make it feel morally easier to keep the rest ('in line with the wishes of the testator'), and the other way round. We also have evidence, as we shall discuss, that keeping money for a while before doing something else with it may serve a number of functions. So, the boundaries between keeping money and doing other things with it are slippery and fluid over time and space but, despite this, keeping or investing money does entail a distinctive set of practices, which we discuss here.

Overall, we have twenty-eight accounts of people keeping or investing inherited money. How people do this varies from putting it into a savings or investment account, buying shares or investing in some other way, starting up a business, or making purchases considered to be 'an investment', most notably houses. We refer to this last as 'investment spending'. We have included examples where people invest money for others (four examples of people investing money for children), and where people keep land and houses (very few examples – land is rarely inherited, and houses are almost always sold, not kept). Some people, like Helena Muhkerjee quoted above, invest in a variety of ways as well as doing other things with it.

Keeping or investing are the most popular things to do with inherited money in our interview data. There is a fairly even distribution of women and men who report doing this, except investing for children (four examples, all female) and keeping land (the three Asian third party examples already referred to, all male). By contrast with our 'giving it away' examples, keeping and investing involve a range of types of bequest (estates, houses, specified cash sums) and a wider range of genealogical relationships of testator to beneficiary (most commonly parent–child but also aunt–niece or nephew, grandparent–grandchild and friend–friend). The sums involved vary from the very small to the very large. What binds these examples together, however, is that they are characterised by a set of practices that are, for the respondents, essentially about keeping, preserving or investing the money they have inherited: these are the kinds of words they use to describe what they have done. Overall, people are telling us that inherited money is special and should not be treated just like any other money. Ruth Jakes, who recently inherited a modest £50 from a friend of her parents, and who invested it jointly with her fiancé in a building society account, explained how she feels:

> It's, like, special ... and yet in a way I don't feel as though it was mine. I don't feel it's mine to spend on me.
> (Ruth Jakes, 18, single, living in family home)

While everyone in these examples is treating inherited money as special, they are not necessarily all trying to achieve the same thing through their actions of investing or keeping the money. So what can be achieved by doing this?

First, the act of investing rather than, for example, using money for routine spending (such as domestic shopping or household expenses) helps to *make money special* – or keep it special – because it is not being treated like 'any old money' and, for some people, because it is something the person who gave it to them would have approved of. Helena Muhkerjee says of her aunt:

> I'd like to think that, you know, if she could be sitting on my shoulder now, she'd be saying 'you did just the right thing'.
> (Helena Muhkerjee, 40s, married, home owner)

Here there is a real sense of recognising that you have been entrusted with something and needing to feel and possibly show that you are worthy of that trust by doing something worthwhile with that thing. This is the kind of sentiment that lies behind the commonly held view expressed above by Ruth Jakes that inherited money is not quite your own, or is more special, more significant, than your own. For some, like Sandra Thompson, this is because it represents 'the sum of someone else's achievements'.

It is in this sense of keeping and making inherited money special that we should understand what 'investment' means, rather than thinking that we are observing some form of economic rationality. There is no sense in our data that people are talking about investing inherited money in terms of economic rationality. For example, no one talks about searching for the best interest rate or of the importance of 'growing' the resource for the sake of the investment principle *per se*. Instead, people seem to be trying to do something *sensible* (again, a word that is often used specifically) with the money and to treat it with respect. That respect involves recognising that it was special enough to the testator for them to mark it out and pass it on to you and, as suggested above, that feeling may be particularly marked where the money was a personalised cash gift ('I give £100 to Susan Smith'), rather than a share of a whole. In a sense, making money special by investing it means that it continues to bear the imprint of the person who has died and your relationship with them, because you have tried your best to think it through from their perspective: that is, what it meant to them, what they would have thought a worthwhile use for it, what they gave it to you for. But, crucially, it is the beneficiary's interpretative moral action that confirms that it is special money. Throughout our data set we get the very strong message that it is inappropriate for testators to try to control how beneficiaries spend their money or use their legacies.

Investing inherited money is not, therefore, governed by an economic rationality but instead by a relational form of moral reasoning. Of course, the options available for investment are socially defined, and seeing investment as a means of 'treating money as special' is undoubtedly culturally derived and has wider social and economic consequences.

A second reason for investing inherited money, especially where this involves putting it into some form of savings or investment account, is that it is a useful holding strategy at a time when a beneficiary may simply not know what to do with the money, or not feel ready to decide. Eventually, the money may be spent or invested in a variety of ways, but what keeping money in this kind of 'holding strategy' way also achieves, very significantly, is the *passing of time*. Gradually, during this time, a sense of ownership – both practical and moral – may be transferred from testator to beneficiary. To paraphrase Ruth Jakes (above), after a while, it may come to seem more like your own money. Investing inherited money can therefore seem a respectable and sensible course of action in the short term, and it can certainly enable beneficiaries to avoid the accusation that they have acted with 'unseemly haste' (which we discuss further below).

Third, all the time during which a beneficiary neither spends nor gives away money, it is 'still there' and in a sense perhaps the person and the relationship whom it symbolises can be felt to be 'still there'. This achieves a sense of respect for the testator, which, we have noted, seems to be an important moral consideration. However, there may also be moral hazards in keeping money 'too long' – not least that a beneficiary might be perceived as 'living in the past'. Beneficiaries may have to weigh up the relative moral risks of retaining or using it.

We have only two clear accounts in our data of people wishing to keep inherited money intact and in perpetuity – literally to preserve it as 'family money' in the sense outlined in Chapter 1. Both are accounts by a husband or wife about their spouse and, in both cases, our respondent is highly critical of what they see as their partner's 'hoarding'. The first of these is Paul Watson, whose late wife had received money from her mother, which had been passed to her intact by her mother and was apparently being passed down the generations of women in her family. His late wife had intended to pass the money to her children (although she had not written this into a will before she died) in accordance with this family tradition and had left it 'untouched' for many years. In fact, Paul inherited the whole of his wife's estate and clearly felt that the principle of keeping money intact for the next generation was at odds with the principle of financial interdependence between spouses, which he felt his wife had contravened. He spent the money, and reasoned that this was morally acceptable because he had financial need and because his wife had failed to use the money at key times in the past when together they had encountered financial difficulties. Essentially, what he was challenging was the notion of 'family money', which is never owned outright by any one individual but is passed intact down the generations. Ironically, perhaps, he was also challenging his wife's right to ownership of money independent of him as her spouse, and we shall return to the question of individual and joint ownership of inherited money shortly.

Although most people do not challenge the notion of family money in quite such a direct fashion, literally by breaking a chain, Paul's sentiments about it are strongly echoed in our data. Almost universally, when asked whether a testator should be able to place restrictions on how their beneficiaries use inherited money, our respondents say no they should not. Although many beneficiaries clearly do not feel free or willing to use inherited money as though it is any other kind of money, there is also strong resistance to the idea that testators should prescribe how it may be used. It is the beneficiary's moral job to realise that the money is special and work out how to use it in a way that best honours and respects the individual who left it to them and their relationship with them. But Paul Watson's account, and that of Rita Dixon, our only other 'family money' example, suggest that the beneficiary's moral reasoning may need to incorporate something of their own current relationships with living relatives, who are certainly likely to form a view about how appropriately they are using their inheritance. Rita Dixon's father inherited £2,000 from his mother seventeen years ago and has kept it intact. Rita is very critical of his 'keeping it to himself', as she puts it, 'because he said that his mother wouldn't want him to touch it'. His mother had been very 'thrifty', but Rita clearly sees his decision not to share around the money now (she says if she inherited she would 'share it amongst the kids') as selfish, even though it is likely she will benefit on his death should she survive him.

The fourth point is that, 'investment spending' is potentially a respectable way of spending inherited money on oneself. For example, one of our respondents, a young man, has spent part of a fairly large inheritance on tools and equipment for his trade, and he talks of this very openly and with some pride as an investment (in himself) for the future. There are, of course, other ways of spending money that have nothing to do with the concept of investment, and it is to these that we now turn.

Spending money

If people are not going to give all their inherited money away, or invest it all, then spending it is the other option. In many ways this is the most problematic of the three. We have thirty-four accounts of people spending inherited money in different ways (not including investment spending). The most interesting feature is not so much what they spend it on as what kind of *spending practice* they use. The relationship between these elements is not always direct. Aside from investment spending, we have identified four other spending practices:

- *Routine spending*, where people spend the money as though it were any other money.
- *Opportunity spending*, where inherited money is treated as giving the opportunity to buy something out of the ordinary for the person or their family – usually spouse or children.
- *Reckless spending*.
- *Commemorative spending*, where money is spent commemoratively in respect of the person who has died.

Routine spending

The most significant point about the first spending practice, routine spending, is that it seems highly unpopular. Routine spending is where people use inherited money as though it were any other money, for example to pay the gas bill, for living expenses, to pay the rent or the mortgage. We have ten examples of this kind of spending, evenly split between men and women. In most cases, these actions are linked overtly to economic need and lack of choice. Most people talk about regretting having to spend the money like this and, for example, wishing they could have invested it. We do have three further examples (all women) where people talk about buying specific utilitarian items, and in two of these cases it is significant that this form of spending is being differentiated from routine spending in rather important ways. Jennifer Murray (and her sister, not interviewed) bought dishwashers with money from their aunt's estate. She points out that this would have gained her aunt's approval and amusement as 'she always washed up at our houses'. Jean Seddon used the cigarette coupons her mother passed to her just before she died to buy an ironing board cover and a purse from the catalogue. She says that the cover arrived on the day her mother died, and the purse arrived the day of the funeral. Both of these accounts are interesting, and differentiated from our other examples of routine spending, in that respondents are able to see a symbolic significance to do with the person who has died in rather utilitarian purchases, and that they feel they have 'something to show for it'. It may be significant that our examples of this all come from women, although the numbers are too small for us to draw any conclusions.

Opportunity spending

This second form of spending practice is where people spend inherited money on things they would not otherwise have. In a sense in spending in this way they are treating the inherited money as though it were both special – because it enables them to have or do something out of the ordinary – and fortuitous. These people are deliberately not using the money routinely, and sometimes they will use it to buy items for their own children. We have five examples of this kind of spending, where money has been used for cars, holidays and, in one case, a honeymoon.

Reckless spending

We suggested earlier that there is a connection between how people spend and what they spend money on, but it is not a one-to-one relationship. Reckless spending – often referred to as 'blowing it' – illustrates this. The cars and holidays that can be viewed as the products of opportunity spending would be seen in other circumstances as spending of a much more reckless kind. Reckless spending stands in direct contrast to investment spending in particular. We have ten examples where, according to our interviewees, beneficiaries of money have 'blown it'. Almost invariably, that is the exact term used. Alternatively, people talk of 'squandering' and 'wasting' money. The legacies in these examples come from a tight range of kin (most commonly parents, then grandparents, and one from a spouse) and involve either whole or part estates, or fairly substantial (in the interviewees' terms) cash gifts. The people who 'blow it' are both women and men, and none of our interviewees of Asian origin figures in these accounts. However, probably the most important point to make here is that the people who 'blow it' are, almost invariably, *other people*. Eight of our ten examples are third party accounts. Few people portray themselves as reckless spenders of inherited money. The only two who did were both young adults. Many of the other accounts suggest that 'blowing it' is something that young people are perceived to be 'at risk' of doing if not suitably reined in. The most common items that people are perceived as having 'blown' money on are cars, holidays and home improvements. It should be noted that all of these items can be bought through other spending practices. Thus it is not the items purchased that makes spending 'reckless' but the context in which the purchases are made.

The term 'blowing it' is used in quite specific ways – mostly to do with horror stories and moral tales involving not doing all the things that investment spending and investment can do: for example, not treating the money as special; not thinking your way into the perspective of the person who has died; spending it too quickly or with unseemly haste; or spending hard-earned money irresponsibly on ephemeral things. For example, Madonna Smith tells us that her father had inherited money from his wife (her mother), which he had spent on a wedding to and honeymoon with his subsequent wife. She says: 'My mother would have gone absolutely mad ... that was money for him ... to look after him'. Clearly, she feels that her father has spent the money in an inappropriate way that fails to honour his relationship with his first wife. This could also be construed as an example of 'money passing out of the family', as discussed in Chapter 2, because the money has been spent on someone who had no personal relationship, and no genetic link, with the testator. Another example of reckless spending comes from Jackie Giles, referring to friends who spent money inherited from parents on home improvements within six months. She says: 'I think I would feel I was spending their life away'. Not only has the money been spent too quickly but also it has been treated with insufficient respect, or as insufficiently special. Similarly, Dorothy Ford's uncle inherited his mother's estate, but he sold everything and spent all the money very quickly and, according to Dorothy, 'he never did a day's work in his life'.

The practice of reckless spending raises in stark form what is nevertheless a theme elsewhere: that beneficiaries' own interpretations of their actions and practices may be at odds with those of people who know them. A beneficiary may have to try to consider, in their moral reasoning, the perspectives not only of themselves and the person who has died but also of others with whom they currently are (and the person who has died may have formerly been) enmeshed in kin relationships. These current relationships may have more to do with their own sets of responsibilities and connections – 'my family' – than those of the testator, yet they are simultaneously trying to balance these against the testator's memory. Our data suggest that people are reluctant to describe themselves as reckless spenders of inherited money, unless they can say they were 'too young to know better'. This adds weight to the idea that people feel that how they spend inherited money is a reflection upon themselves and the value they give to their kin relationships, past and present.

Commemorative spending

By contrast with reckless spending, commemorative spending is highly respectable, and accounts tend to come from the actors themselves. We had six examples (all women, although some men were mentioned as siblings doing the same thing) of people engaging explicitly in commemorative spending, which means that they have used inherited money to buy something specifically as a memento of the person who died. In a sense, they are creating their own keepsake to carry the memory of that person (see Chapter 6 for a discussion of keepsakes and symbolism). The types of inherited gift that our respondents used in this way varied from whole estates through to large and very small cash gifts received from aunts and uncles, a mother, friends, a brother and a grandmother.

For example, Ellen Beech bought an emerald ring with money from her aunt but had in mind that her daughter would like the ring, so she could pass it on to her when she died. Betty Hill and her siblings bought a commemorative tree with part of the proceeds of the sale of her mother's possessions. Meg Russell bought a picture of the Lake District to 'remember' her uncle by.

For some people, commemorative spending is clearly a way of dealing with the morally problematic nature of clearing a house and selling *en masse* the possessions of someone who has died. For others, it is about creating some form of embodiment – as a keepsake – of that person and of the relationship they had with them.

Individual and joint ownership of inherited money

So far in this chapter, we have discussed beneficiaries as *individuals*, but most of the people in our study who had inherited money were married at the time when they received the legacy. This raises the important question of whether beneficiaries think and act as individuals or jointly in their use of the money they have inherited. We have twenty-four examples of people talking about this, most involving examples where one partner has been a beneficiary in the past, and a few where people have responded to a question about whether they would regard any money inherited in the future as joint or individual. Over two-thirds of these (seventeen) say that money was or would be shared between partners, while the remainder (seven) say that the money belongs to one or other partner. Here are some examples of people talking about sharing inherited money:

HUGH DALTON: It went into the general pool ... We've always pooled our resources.
SYLVIA DALTON: It's always been one purse.
(70s and 60s, married, privately rented sheltered accommodation; speaking of inherited money from both of their sets of parents)

We shared it. We've got one of those families where nothing is anybody's, everything is everybody's.
(Wendy Khan, 40s, married, home owner; regarding money inherited from her parents)

You generally get it when you don't really need it ... I don't know what we'd do, you know. I mean the car's all right now. We go on holiday every year. Other than going on holiday twice a year, I couldn't go twice a year on holiday I don't think, our kids, well they wouldn't be kids then, they'd be, our children would be struggling to make ends meet or living in a one-roomed bedsit or whatever ... So I would definitely put it into some sort of house for them, you know. Something that's going to be of value ... houses, you know, they tend to keep their value. It would be joint, me and Jackie [wife] I wouldn't think of keeping it all for myself and saying 'Oh I'll have a new suit (laughs) and I'll buy myself a new car and you can have your old banger like'. No I would see it as joint money. But we have always done that, me and Jackie.

(Eddie Giles, 30s, married, home owner; speculating on what he would do if he should inherit money from his parents)

Most people used the opportunity of talking to us about inheriting money to make general statements of this kind about the quality of family or marriage they had (equal, fair, sharing, co-operative), and to link what they did with inherited money with their way of organising money in general. The idea of spending some money on children occurs commonly, particularly in the examples where people are being asked to speculate on what they would do should they inherit some money from a relative. However, it does not seem that children – of any age – had a joint *say* in how the money was used. But sharing inherited money between partners does not always mean joint ownership and control of the money either. We get the sense in many of the accounts that the person who is the beneficiary is recognised to be making a *choice* to share their inheritance, and in doing so it is made apparent that the money is theirs – individually – to make choices about. The very fact that so many make the choice to 'share' the money is significant. It tells us that the webs of family relationships and responsibilities in which people are currently enmeshed provide an important context within which decisions are made about using inherited money. As Eddie Giles so eloquently puts it, people are unlikely to feel able or willing to keep money 'to themselves' in a context where those with whom they share finances, or for whom they feel responsible, do not derive some benefit.

Sharing inherited money with a partner does help people to establish to themselves and others that they are not selfish, and that they are tuned into the needs and sensibilities of the living as well as to the memory of the dead. This seems highly important to our respondents, and significantly it is also a dominant theme in our seven examples where people talk about individual rather than joint control of inherited money, such as in the case of Mavis Douglas.

MAVIS: It was my money. I actually spent it in the house ... which is how we both benefited from it. But Ken wouldn't let me put it in [their joint account], he said I had to have it as my own, you know. But I spent it in the house.
INTERVIEWER: And was it you who decided how to spend it?
MAVIS: Oh yes. I decided that ... I put it away until I thought about things, you know, and then spent it.
INTERVIEWER: Why did you spend it on the house and not on yourself?
MAVIS: Um, well, so everyone got the benefit of it. It would have been rather selfish, really, and it gave me pleasure doing that. Cos we've sort of always had to struggle.
(Mavis Douglas, 50s, second marriage, home owner; talking about money inherited from her parents)

This account helps to illustrate some of the ambiguities about joint and individual money, because although Mavis is clear that the money was *her* money, she also uses her account to establish that it was only hers because her husband insisted that it be so and, in the event, she spent it on something from which he and her children could benefit. It is significant both that the ways in which Mavis used *her* money do not look individually determined and that she gives a rationale for her actions that draws heavily on and constructs a self-identity as an *unselfish beneficiary*.

We think this is more than an example of the general tendency for women to spend money of any derivation on their households rather than on themselves (Vogler and Pahl 1994). We have no examples of individuals – male or female – who are part of a couple but who spent money entirely on themselves, although some of those who talk of sharing the money also mention buying some small things for themselves (clothes, for example). The only two cases we have of the money not being shared with the spouse in some way are the third party examples given by Paul Watson and Rita Dixon, which we discussed earlier. These both involved partners preserving money that they had inherited from a parent and, as discussed, both had been open to criticism for 'hoarding' money that they (according to our respondent) should have shared and spent. Here is Paul Watson's example. He is talking about his deceased wife:

> Mary's mother left it to Mary and Mary got it. Mary was thinking about leaving it to the children and I disagree. I think that's wrong because I worked all my life to pay for everything. Elaine worked a bit of the time, but I mean my cash went to bringing the family up and providing a home. And let's face it, I mean I can't – if I were in that position – I can't sell the home I live in can I for the cash to live by? Whereas if I'd have died Mary would have got the house plus her own cash. Plus Mary would have got a pension which I don't get and I think ... that sort of thing's a bit unfair.
> (Paul Watson, 50s, cohabiting, home owner)

We can identify the gendered view of the ways in which women and men contribute to the household economy that Paul provides in several of our other accounts (including Mavis Douglas above), and it is likely that the 'right' of a beneficiary to keep and dispose of inherited money in individually determined ways may be circumscribed where it is perceived that they have contributed less in financial terms to the household than their partner. However, as mentioned we do not see that right frequently exercised in any case. What is particularly significant about Paul Watson's account is his objection to the idea that money should be preserved intact when it is needed (by spouse and household) during the owner's lifetime. He is making the point very strongly that current responsibilities (especially those to a spouse) should take precedence over the principle of 'family money', which he clearly holds in some contempt. In his case, his wife did keep the money during her lifetime, although we suspect that she would have seen herself more as a trustee of family money – since she had preserved it throughout times of economic need – than an individual owner of it, and would have contested his description of it as 'her own cash'.

Nevertheless, Paul's wife was open to his criticism (as was Rita Dixon's husband) of being selfish largely because the notion of family money is a less current and potent inheritance discourse than is the idea that you are selfish if you do not use inherited money, at least in part, for the benefit of your spouse and household. Beneficiaries are simultaneously having to operate as individuals who are connected to a specific individual testator, now deceased, and as part of a couple (and sometimes household). The tensions that can result are most starkly expressed in extreme cases, where the 'family property' view of money and the 'spend it now where it's needed' view most clearly collide. This requires a beneficiary to face the question of whether she or he should give priority to the living or to the dead. This brings the tension between present and past relationships into sharp focus. But underlying all of the examples is a process whereby a beneficiary is operating at the interface between past and present, balancing the needs and sensibilities of some of the living ('my family') with the memory of one of the dead (and their version of 'my family').

Conclusion

Receiving money as part or all of an inheritance is not easy or straightforward. Inherited money is 'difficult money', and for many beneficiaries working out what to do with it has to be done in the midst of profound grief and loss. Inherited money is not necessarily difficult because it is *money*, however. Our data on other forms of inheritance, and particularly on 'keepsakes', demonstrates moral difficulties there too (see Chapter 6). Instead, we are led to the conclusion that these 'transactions' of inheritance are not tricky because money is involved *per se* but because *kin relationships* – past, present and future – are involved. Inheriting money requires the beneficiary to make decisions about what to do with it, but our arguments suggest that these become active *moral* decisions precisely because they are about, and made within, relationships that operate over time. In that sense, people use money to fashion their own moralities of kinship in relational ways.

Becoming a beneficiary means that you are entrusted with a moral responsibility in relation to the assets themselves, to the person who has died, and to others with whom you and they had and have relationships. But you are not given a clear prescription or set of rules about how to proceed. As we have suggested, people see it as entirely inappropriate for testators to try to provide such a prescription, even though many are not averse to making moral judgements about how beneficiaries actually do use money. The job of working out what to do potentially involves a range of practices and forms of reasoning: commemorative, relational, personal and practical, and it involves thinking about 'family' across time, from past to present to future. In this chapter, we have seen that people do this by reasoning about:

- *What is inherited.* That is, the type of gift – cash, a part estate, and so on.
- *What it represents.* For example 'the sum of someone else's achievements', or something special that is 'not quite mine to spend on me'.
- *Its economic value.*
- *Who gave the gift.* Genealogy seems less significant here than the beneficiary's relationship with the person who has died, what they think their intentions might have been, what they might have approved of, and what action the beneficiary thinks will best help them to commemorate that person. The demeanour and actions associated with receiving (how gracious, how genuine the thanks, how quickly forgotten, and so on) all say something about the value that the recipient places on the donor. For beneficiaries of an inheritance, however, this moral etiquette becomes much more complex because the physical presence of the donor is removed.
- *What other people have inherited* (or have not inherited), including a consideration of their genealogical position, their relationship to the testator (its quality, history) and their needs. In part, this expresses the testator's view of 'my inheritance family', which the beneficiary now has to reconcile with their own view of 'my family'.
- *Current relationships and commitments* ('my family') and how these are influenced by this inheritance. In particular, people feel a pull between those who are part of their own current domestic economy and the testator's version of 'my family'.
- *Oneself and one's own identity*, for example, 'the unselfish beneficiary'), and one's own economic and other circumstances.

In these ways, through the work and interpretative actions of beneficiaries, inherited money comes to symbolise a point of connection (sometimes a tension) between the 'my family' of the testator and the beneficiary, and between a past and a present (or pasts and presents) in family lives. Simultaneously, moralities of spending, consuming and owning money inherited from a relative are crafted. It is easy for beneficiaries to get it wrong, and to 'sin' while traversing this difficult terrain, with so many potential critics of one's actions and motives. The first of these critics is the beneficiary him or herself, in their reflexive view of their own actions and the kind of self-identity they wish to create. Second are others, especially but not only other kin, and their judgements about how the beneficiary has handled things. Third is the person who has died both in the form of the beneficiary's memory and commemoration of them but also in the possibility that their spirit is, as Helena Muhkerjee put it, 'sitting on your shoulder'.

That inheriting money requires beneficiaries to make decisions that are morally difficult points to an important underlying issue. This is that beneficiaries do not see inherited money as a normal or routine part of their own lifestyle or domestic economy. If it were, then people would have less difficulty in deciding how it should be spent. This underlines very clearly a point that surfaces again and again in our data: that people do not have a right to expect an inheritance. We think that what people are telling us is that inheritance of money is a *bonus*, not a *necessity*. This raises questions about what ownership of property means across generations in families, which we address directly in the following chapter.

Chapter 5

Questions of ownership

Introduction

In the previous chapter, we considered what people do with inherited money and what this tells us about morality in the inheritance process. In turn, this raised some questions about the nature of property ownership. Our data suggested that beneficiaries see inherited property as a bonus rather than an automatic right. Even those who are children of the deceased do not appear to see themselves as 'owners in waiting' of their parents' property.

However, this picture is only partial, since the last chapter concentrated simply on the perspective of those who had received money. In this chapter, we shall broaden our focus to include those who are the donors (actual and potential) as well as the recipients in the inheritance process. We shall still concentrate upon the transmission of major assets – houses, land, money – leaving to the next chapter a discussion of the inheritance of personal property.

In this chapter, therefore, we are drawing together the various strands of our discussion on property 'ownership' and, in particular, whether there is any sense in which 'the family' is the owner. By this we mean an understanding that each generation has a responsibility to retain property and to pass it on – intact or possibly enhanced – to the next. Thus no individual has full and moral ownership of the property, whatever the legal position. In such a system, the property is 'owned' transgenerationally. It is family property, in a strong sense.

Is there any evidence in our data that English families do regard property as transgenerationally owned? This is the key question to be explored in this chapter. In the process, we uncover not only the nature of property ownership but also more insights into the nature of kinship. For example, do people use ownership of property to constitute kin relationships, and if so, in what ways? And conversely, how do kin relationships influence what ownership itself can and does mean in the inheritance process?

Financing old age: a 'case study'

We begin with a 'case study' to explore questions of ownership, namely financing old age. In particular, we consider the question of whether older people and their families are prepared to contemplate the use of assets – most commonly a house – to finance personal care and support when needed.

This is a fruitful focus for exploring questions of ownership in the sense outlined above. For example, it raises questions about whether elderly people do, or should try to, preserve (or even generate) assets to pass on via inheritance, or whether it is legitimate to 'spend it before you go' on the basis that your property is yours and 'you can't take it with you'. This means that the whole question of whether or not there is anything left to be passed on is likely to be raised in stark form, and issues about whether or not anything *should* be left are likely to be at the forefront in people's processes of reasoning about these matters. The specific case of financing old age therefore provides a window on questions of family property and transgenerational ownership.

Financing old age: a narrative

We begin our discussion with a narrative. As we explained in Chapter 2, where we first introduced the narrative as an analytical device, this is a composite story constructed from common themes in accounts given by interviewees. Here, as there, the scenarios developed in the narrative are those our interviewees worry about, or disapprove of, or wish to avoid. They are based on a combination of interviewees' own experiences, the experiences of others known to them, and their comments about situations of which they approve and disapprove. The different variations on the narrative go like this:

Main narrative
Anita is an elderly widowed home owner, with a small pension and modest savings. She has three adult children, all married, with children. She knows that circumstances may arise where she may have to choose between her own needs and preserving enough money to pass on after she dies.

Variation 1
1 Anita becomes ill and needs personal care.
2 She moves into a residential care home nearby but wants to keep her house in case her health improves and she is able to go home. She uses her savings to pay the fees.
3 Anita's health doesn't improve. Some time later, she runs out of money. She is required to sell her house so that she can continue to pay the fees.
4 Some years later, Anita dies. The proceeds from her house sale and her savings have nearly all been used to pay the fees.
5 Her children inherit her remaining personal possessions, but no assets or money.

The main issue in this variation is an element of 'official compulsion': an elderly person of limited means is obliged to sell her house and use her savings to pay for care. As a consequence, she has nothing left to pass on to her children.

Variation 2
1 Anita becomes increasingly frail but continues to manage living alone. She is very careful with money and spends little on herself.
2 Anita's neighbour helps when she can but thinks that Anita 'scrimps and saves' too much. She advises Anita to use some of her money to make life easier: to pay for regular help at home, to eat better, and to keep the house warmer.
3 Anita doesn't take her neighbour's advice and continues to live frugally on her pension, without touching her savings. She wants to make sure her children have something to inherit when she dies.
4 Some years later, Anita dies. Her children inherit her estate.

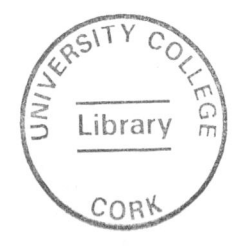

In this variation, the core theme is that an elderly person denies her own needs in order to provide for adult children through inheritance.

Variation 3
1 Anita is fairly fit and healthy but has little money available to spend and would like some help in the home.
2 She decides to release some of the equity in her house to pay for home help and so that she can live in a little more comfort. She enters into an equity release scheme with a commercial financial institution. In return for a small cash sum and a regular income, together with the right to stay in her home for the rest of her life, Anita transfers ownership of her house to that institution.
3 Six months later, Anita dies. She has spent most of the cash sum, and the regular income ceases on her death. Her children inherit her remaining personal possessions, and a small amount of cash.

In this variation, the core issue is the ultimate consequences of an equity release scheme: a commercial financial institution profits from Anita's circumstances. As a consequence, she has nothing left to pass on to her children.

Although we have produced a composite version, references to this narrative, with its different variations, occur in the accounts of seventy-seven of our interviewees (forty-nine women and twenty-eight men), 80 per cent of our total, most of whom we had asked directly about these issues. Nearly all of these seventy-seven provide accounts that can be categorised wholly or partly as one or more of the variations given above. This suggests that in our study the vast majority of people recognise and identify with this narrative, whether or not it actually reflects their own experience.

Using money and assets in old age

The narrative above centres on questions about the use of money and assets in old age, and the role of kinship and inheritance in that process. What does it tell us about the questions of ownership, inheritance and kinship with which we began this chapter? We can explore this best by drawing upon our interview data.

The first and most important point, and the one that in a sense subsumes all the rest, is that *elderly people have an inalienable right to use their money as they wish*, whatever that may entail. This theme surfaces in a number of ways and contexts that we shall consider, some of which are touched on in the reasoning of one of our interviewees about equity release schemes:

> Providing I could keep my head above water type of thing, I'd prefer the house to be mine, not belonging to somebody else virtually. I'd much prefer, you know, then it could be passed on to the family ... but I don't think they've any *right* to it, but that's the way I would like it to be ... Because this [house] is mine, it's nobody else's.
> (David Bailey, 60s, married, home owner)

David's view, echoed by many others in our study, is that his house belongs to him, not his family, and not an insurance company or bank, as long as he can help it. He is asserting his right to use and dispose of his property as he wishes. It so happens that he would like to pass on the full value of his house to his children, but this is not the main point of his comments. He emphasises very clearly that his children should not have the house as of right. David Bailey's comments articulate the view that elderly people have a right to spend or save money as they choose. Giving absolute priority to the personal choice of the elderly person allows for the possibility that some may *choose* to use their money to pay for care. The message that comes through clearly from our data is that if elderly people *wish* to use their money to pay for care rather than to preserve it for children or relatives, then this is acceptable. Karen Horn sees it as a matter of right that people should be able to sell their homes to pay for care. Others, especially those who have professional experience of dealing with elderly people and their relatives in some form or other, like Dorothy Ford and Souresh Khan, are critical of what they see as relatives 'crawling out of the woodwork', as Dorothy puts it, to try to prevent elderly people using their assets in this way. Again, the rights of elderly people to make their own decisions about money and assets are strongly asserted by our interviewees. No one suggested otherwise.

That does not mean, however, that people generally approve of the principle of paying for care, or that the desire to have 'something to leave' one's own children is absent. These are the issues dealt with in Variation 1 of our narrative above. While some interviewees do approve of paying for care ('they're not going to spend it on anything else are they?' says Doris Clegg), others, especially those for whom this is a current or recent preoccupation in their own lives, say that elderly people should not *have to* do this, or that they should not have to pay so much. Phoebe Rogers argued that the state should pay for care, so that elderly people can choose whether to keep their money, spend it on something 'wacky or wild', or pass it on to their children. Sylvia Dalton felt that the costs were so high that such choices were effectively removed:

> You feel we've saved, well I think we have, and we've taken things easy and not gone daft spending and what have you, and so at the end of the day you like to think there's something for your family ... and if you have to go into a home, well of course, I assume you have to pay if you've to go into a home. But it seems to be taking *everything*. They could be taking everything off you and leaving your family with nothing ... This is the only thing that is in the back of your mind, and you feel you'd like to do something about it before it all goes.
> (Sylvia Dalton, 60s, married, first-generation home owner; emphasis in original)

Aloisious Lovejoy put it more strongly:

> I've not worked all my life to give my money back to the ruddy government ... You've worked all your life and paid your national contributions, your national health stamp, and then they want to make you pay for being ill ... If you have any possessions you pass it on to your children, don't you?
> (Aloisious Lovejoy, 80s, first-generation home owner)

The strongest theme is a reaction against the 'official compulsion', which has the effect of *removing the inherent right to choice* from the elderly person. Part of the reasoning here is that assets are the sum of a lifetime's effort. The government should have no claim upon them, because they have been earned, especially when taxes and National Insurance contributions have already been paid.

This money has come from lots of small and large daily endeavours, decisions and personal economies. *It is highly personal.* It may be tied up now in the capital value of the home that the person is living in, but in no sense is it a common resource that the state or others have a right to draw upon. It is not that kind of money.

The idea that elderly people's money is personal because it is the sum of their lifetime's effort was expressed strongly and frequently by our interviewees, including one who said that 'we've always earned every penny we've got' despite having received a sizeable bequest from an aunt. Nevertheless, that money had been earned, originally, and given our discussion in the previous chapter about the relational nature of the use of money, it is perhaps unsurprising that our interviewee would see this as 'her own' money, rather than view it as a common resource.

So part of the reaction against 'official compulsion' rests upon a sense that money is highly personal. This is reinforced by our interviewees' reasoning concerning the *role of the state in social welfare.* For some, this is quite straightforward. The state should pay for care. It is not fair that people should have to 'pay for being ill', as Aloisious Lovejoy put it, when whether or not elderly people have good or poor health is a bit of a lottery. Daisy Taylor said: 'I think the state has enough money'. Sandra Fisher said: 'why should the state have it when she's [mother] never claimed anything from the state in her life?' For others, it is not so clearcut and is further complicated by considerations about who is deserving of state help and who is not. Several people talked about the injustice of someone who has saved all their life having to use that money to pay for care, when the person 'in the next bed', or 'in the next room', who by implication had not been so careful, got the same level of care free.

There were even more ambiguities and contradictions for some people. Howard Kent used his interview to think through some of these. Talking of a friend's current situation, he said:

> People who have squandered their money, they can go out drinking and smoking and they expect, I don't know the rights and wrongs of it, but they go into these homes and everything's paid for them and they get about £10 pocket money some of them. And somebody else who, like this man [his friend], they've got to pay their own way ... I feel it's unfair,

but at the same time I don't see why the government should pay for someone for him to leave it to somebody who, you know, hasn't done anything for him ... Why should the government pay for him to be in this home so that he can leave his money to somebody that really, in my opinion, doesn't deserve it.

(Howard Kent, 50s, single, first-generation home owner)

Howard's dilemma rather nicely encapsulates our main points about paying for care. Essentially, most of our interviewees are saying that elderly people should not have their rights to use their property in whatever way they choose removed: by the state, if they want to leave it to relatives; or by relatives, if they want to pay for their own care. Complications arise in cases like Howard's, however, where both relatives and the state are seen to be making illegitimate claims. What really irks Howard is that his friend's son (and possibly his friend himself) are treating the money as family money, transgenerationally owned, where the son is already seen as an owner in waiting. He regards that as objectionable.

That they should not *have to* pay for care, or *have to* leave their money to relatives, underpins a very prominent theme in our data, that is that elderly people have a *right to a comfortable life, financial security and dignity*. For some, this extends to a right to have fun (spending money on something 'wacky and wild'). Sometimes, this is counterposed to a 'grasping' state or unscrupulous private care homes, which would take all the money given a chance. Annie Palfrey sums this up:

> I think there should be some means of at least giving them some dignity, some savings, some money. Not taking it all.
>
> (Annie Palfrey, 50s, single, privately rented accommodation)

In eight cases, either our interviewee or a close relative had considered taking action to try to divert assets to their adult children as a way of avoiding having to use them to pay for care. They all felt forced into considering this (by a 'grasping' state) and hence that such action might be morally justifiable. But people were uncomfortable about it for a different reason: the loss of financial independence and of dignity. As one interviewee said of a parent, 'she doesn't want to come and ask us for money'.

An elderly person loses dignity when a grasping state obliges him or her to forgo control of personal assets in order to receive care, which really should be financed by the tax payer. This is a strong image in our data. Even more common, however, is the loss of dignity that flows from 'scrimping and saving', denying one's own needs, leading an impoverished existence, in order to pass money on to one's children as in Variation 2 of our narrative above. This image was sometimes constructed in relation to third parties (like Howard Kent's friend). More often, however, it emerged in strong statements from interviewees looking 'up' the generations. The adult children of elderly people often said that they did not or would not expect their parents to act in this way. Also, when our interviewees talked about their own old age, this was a frequent theme.

The point is that the image of 'scrimping and saving' is one of which people disapprove, and from which they want to distance themselves and their own family practice. Here are some examples from the data:

> The people that you leave it to will only go and spend it anyway won't they so I don't think you should stint yourself with that thought in mind. I think you should look after yourself first, and then if there's anything left, fair enough [it can go to children].
> (Mavis Douglas, 50s, second marriage, home owner)

> I used to say to mother, don't worry about leaving us anything Mum, please, you know, enjoy yourself.
> (Doris Clegg, 70s, married, privately rented sheltered accommodation)

> If it was my Mum and Dad and they had money and I couldn't take them, I would rather they used what money they had and were well looked after rather than struggle on their own and leave the money ... I think everybody should end their days properly really, not just struggling away on their own.
> (Jackie Giles, 30s, married, home owner)

> If we do accumulate any money as we get older I'd like to think that [my husband] and I could enjoy that together

before we go rather than hand it on to [the children]. I mean I'd like to think I could leave them something but I wouldn't like to think that they were going to be relying on us to be leaving them vast amounts of money and, plus, I think that when we've worked all our lives really, that's not really what it should be for. I feel that we should be able to benefit from it ourselves when we're still young enough to enjoy it.
(Sarah Henderson, 40s, married, first-generation home owner)

I would be the first person to say [to parents] 'For God's sake, go and do it, enjoy yourself, you can't take it with you … think about yourselves first, enjoy the rest of your life, and if there's something left over after you've gone, well aren't we all lucky, but for God's sake don't scrimp and go through all this hardship to leave me something later on when, all being well, I won't need it anyway'. But I've got very deep reservations about it [equity release]. I mean personally I would never want to do it myself. When I die [I would want to know] that at least to begin with they've got what they need and they make of it what they will.
(Helena Muhkerjee, 40s, married, home owner)

Helena Muhkerjee's use of the words 'if there's something left over after you've gone' is echoed in many of our interviewees' accounts. This phrase encapsulates the desirable state of affairs, and the emphasis is upon the 'if'. Older people should not deny their own needs. It is only if a person has lived a comfortable old age and still has some resources – literally, resources that were surplus to her requirements – that there should be anything to pass on. Retaining one's dignity through a comfortable life in old age is the first priority.

One way in which comfort in old age can be secured is through *equity release schemes*, the subject of Variation 3 of our narrative above. They might be said to involve a conscious choice on the part of the elderly person to raise cash against the value of assets, thus also respecting the rights of older people to retain control over these decisions.

However, it turns out that this is by no means a desirable option in the eyes of most of our interviewees who comment on it. There is a variety of equity release schemes and providers on the market (see Davey 1996a, b), but most of our interviewees knew very little about them. Only two had any direct experience of such schemes: one, an interviewee, Peggy Stevenson (widowed, aged 75), who had entered into such a scheme to raise some cash against part of the value of her house; and another whose mother-in-law had done the same. Both had adult children who had been encouraging. The children had emphasised that their parents were free to spend their own money as they wished, and that anyway they themselves were not in financial need. Their parent should therefore feel fully entitled to use their capital to get themselves a decent income.

For the rest of our interviewees, the majority viewed equity release with great suspicion because of what they judged to be high financial risks and the involvement of unscrupulous providers. This view for many had been fuelled by the recent televising of a programme about one particularly unscrupulous provider. Ken Douglas, for example, said that these schemes only seemed advantageous to the banks, and he was very keen that the bank should not get 'their grubby hands on it' (his money). David Bailey, with whom we began our discussion of financing old age, expressed the sentiments of many when he said 'I'd prefer the house to be mine, not belonging to somebody else virtually' and pointed out that he was 'not that desperate'.

Again, then, the themes that emerge are to do with elderly people's dignity, rights to self-determination and control over their own money and assets. Added to this is strong disapproval of commercial organisations, which are seen to be making a profit out of elderly people's need for cash. This, we suspect, is the key to the problem with equity release for our interviewees. The objection is not that elderly people should be able to release some cash for their own use from their assets (rather than preserve it all to pass on to relatives). Rather, it is that the assets pass to a financial institution in return for releasing that cash. This raises the problem of dignity in a different form: the elderly person has to suffer the indignity of becoming indebted.

One might have expected a distinction to be made between elderly people with children (where equity release would be a problem because it removes the children's inheritance) and those without surviving children (where this problem does not arise). However, we find no evidence of such a distinction in our data. As already noted, our two cases of direct experience of equity release both actually involved people with children. Without exception, those interviewees without children who commented on equity release expressed negative views, so although others might have seen equity schemes as potentially suitable for them, they did not. There is no obvious pattern that would distinguish between those with or without children. This is consistent with Davey's study of equity release as an option for older home owners. She found that just over half of the equity release clients in her sample had children, and that it was likely that people with children were *over-* not under-represented in the equity release population more generally (Davey 1996a: 36). Therefore, having children does not, in itself, seem to be a strong barrier to equity release. This does strongly suggest that children are not viewed as 'owners in waiting' of their parents' property.

We therefore conclude that resistance to equity release is normally for reasons other than children's interests. Although our data of themselves would not permit us to make such a generalisation, our conclusion is supported by Davey's evidence, which suggests that attitudes towards inheritance are just one element in a much wider range of explanations for the very limited take-up of equity release among older people. The other explanations involve suspicion, fear of indebtedness or misgivings about government policy directions, all of which, as we have shown, have strong resonance in our data (Davey 1996b).

To sum up so far, our evidence on the use of money in old age points to a number of factors. It points to the inalienable rights of elderly people to use their money as they wish and a deep suspicion of those who would try to modify this: the state, relatives, commercial organisations. The only examples we have of relatives expressing a wish to 'interfere' in what elderly people do with their money involves children saying that parents should *not* save money so that they can pass it on if that means going short themselves in the process. The right to keep control of one's own assets is essential to preserve dignity to the end of one's life. Our evidence also points to a strong view that elderly people's money and assets not only belong to them but are also highly personal possessions with a deeply ingrained symbolic meaning as the expression of a lifetime's economic (in a broad sense) endeavour. It points to a view that property is generationally, not transgenerationally, owned.

Inheritance and parenting

What does this case study of financing old age tell us more generally about inheritance, and about the kin relationships that it both reflects and moulds? In answering these questions, we think it useful to focus on the relationship between inheritance and people's ideas about parenting and how it should be done.

Ideas about parenting are often at the core of what our interviewees are saying. Essentially, many people use the set of questions around financing old age and inheritance, which may or may not have arisen in concrete form in their own lives, as a way of establishing what kind of parent and/or child they are. Their own intentions and practices in relation to assets and money in the inheritance process become part of their way of being a good son or daughter, or a good mother or father, and more generally a key way of expressing and activating a philosophy of parent–child relationships.

The independence of adult children lies at the heart of this. We have already given examples where people told us that they did not expect their parents to leave them anything but, as Helena Muhkerjee put it to her parents, 'if there's something left over after you've gone, well aren't we all lucky'. This expresses a philosophy that adult children should be able to be independent of their parents; they should not rely on receiving an inheritance, but if they do receive one, then this is a bonus. Where the person expressing this sentiment is positioned as the adult child in a parenting relationship, then effectively they are using their approach to questions of ownership and inheritance to say 'yes, I am independent of my parents'. It is clear that, from this perspective, to calculate or expect an inheritance would be strongly disapproved of, as would the notion of transgenerational ownership of family property.

However, most of the comments that our interviewees made about parenting were those in which they were positioned as parents. Two different philosophies, both of which make claims about good parenting, are in operation here. The first says that good parenting involves passing on *something* (if you have something) to your children through inheritance. The second says that good parenting involves instilling the virtues of hard work and independence in your children, and that might involve passing on nothing – it certainly involves making sure that you do not pass on *too much*. Here are some examples of each of these philosophies.

Good parenting involves passing something on

> You're under an obligation, really, to see the family are all right ... It's progress isn't it? You like to think you'd do more for your own children than your parents did for you.
> (Fred Blake, 70s, married, first-generation home owner)

> I've always felt that you've got to leave a little bit.
> (Betty Hill, late 50s, widowed, council rented accommodation)

> No way would I have done that [equity release] ... because I want my kids to have something at the end of the day. This is what it's all about.
> (Mollie Avenham, 70s, widowed, local authority rented accommodation, previously a home owner)

> Within the English community the family is not very strong. I think what happens is once you come of age you leave your parents, do your own thing, work or whatever. And the son goes somewhere else, the daughters get married or whatever, and you never really go back to your parents ... I think they're justified in borrowing money against a house or whatever and living life the way they want to live it because they don't really get back anything from their sons and daughters anyway ... Within our community, I wouldn't have thought so. Why? Because as I said, after a certain time it's the sons who start looking after the parents, you know in their old age ... if then the parents borrowed money against the estate and spent it on themselves and forgot about the son who has looked after them, then it's not justified. Question of ethics.
> (Nazrul Mumtaz, 30s, married, home owner)

Good parenting involves not passing on too much

> I don't think they [parents, in general] owe their children anything at all ... If you've brought them up to the best of

your ability and never seen them short ... I think really you should consider yourself, because they have their life to make some money or do whatever they want. And by the same token, I wouldn't expect them if they went on to big things, I don't automatically think that they should give you their money, you know ... I don't think it should be expected. I think it's just a treat.

(Josie Lewis, 40s, married, first-generation home owner)

Experience is something that you can pass on, and if you can help the children along during the time of your living, fine, but you have to live, at the end of the day, you can't stop living comfortably thinking 'Oh I'll save two pounds today by not eating' and such a thing 'so that my son can have it as an inheritance'. I think that's wrong ... if you want to go on holidays and if there is tied up money [in your house] which can help you know, I won't be reluctant in doing that ... And whatever is left, then they can have it. If there isn't anything left, I am sorry. But ... education is something that I feel very strongly about. I've given them all the opportunity that they can have and once they've had that education they can go on and do what they have to do.

(Souresh Khan, 40s, married, home owner)

I don't see why you should have to limit your spending, you know, money that's yours, just so you can leave it to your children ... If they want a nice comfortable lifestyle they should go out and earn it and, you know, then they deserve it.

(Marianne Horner, 20s, married, home owner)

I think the most important thing with your children is preparing them to make their own way in the world and to fend for themselves and create a good living for themselves ... not to make things, you know, set up an easy life for them.

(Richard Murray, 50s, second marriage, home owner)

I still think that it would be good for my children to make their own way. They shouldn't be helped too much, shouldn't expect too much ... It sounds a bit reactionary, this. But it does build your character. I think that they shouldn't have things too easily ... I don't really assume that I've got to hand on the wealth that we will have to the children ... it's probably better for me if I use some of it before I go, and probably better for them in some way that they should make their own way.

(Greg Henderson, 40s, married, first-generation home owner)

In a sense, these philosophies are not so different. Each concerns how parents and children should handle questions of financial interdependence.

The examples of the philosophy that good parenting involves passing something on do not refer to passing *everything* on. Terms like 'something' or 'a little bit' are used, suggesting that some judgement, some discretion, some restraint should be shown; that passing on 'everything' or 'a lot' might be too much. Therefore, even this philosophy is unlikely to underpin a strong view of family property or transgenerational ownership.

The examples of the philosophy that good parenting involves not passing on too much tend to tie bequeathing in with other elements of parent–child relationships. So, for example, it is all right not to leave anything as long as you have done your best for your children earlier in life: given them a good start. Those other ways of giving children a good start – experience, education, fostering independence – are not only better than money but may even be jeopardised by giving money. Overall, with this philosophy, there is a sense in which it is not good for children to expect inheritance and, moreover, there is the implication that you would have failed as a parent if your child did so.

We might expect those who have never themselves inherited property, or who do not have a family history of owning or thinking about the disposition of property, to see good parenting as instilling virtues of hard work and independence rather than providing material wealth for one's children. Not only would this probably more accurately reflect their own life experience but they also would not have had to deal with the question of what to do with accumulated wealth. Greg Henderson acknowledges this:

Things are very different for us because we are going to hand on a considerable amount of property. Not that it's unique. Lots and lots of people now, most of them do own houses, are going to hand them on, aren't they? But we are the first generation to do it, from the social class we come from. In the past, it hasn't been part of the perception of our parents to worry about wills, because there was nothing to pass on.

(Greg Henderson, 40s, married, first-generation home owner)

Twenty-two of our seventy-five home owners (treating couples as two individuals) are first-generation home owners. The remainder told us that at the very least one or both of their parents had owned property. Certainly, some of the strongest statements of the philosophy that good parenting involves not passing on too much, or indeed anything in a material sense, come from first-generation home owners. However, some of these, like Fred Blake quoted above, draw the opposite conclusion. They want to do more for their children in terms of material inheritance than their parents were able to do for them. Furthermore, and perhaps more significantly, second-generation home owners subscribe to both philosophies. This means that it is not simply the newness of the experience of owning property that creates a view that children should not be given too much in a material sense. If it were, then it might be reasonable to argue that once the spread of housing wealth has filtered down a few generations, this philosophy might give way to the one which says that good parenting involves passing something on. However, our evidence does not support that suggestion.

What is particularly significant for our discussion of ownership and inheritance is that people's understandings of what ownership means, and how inheritance should be handled in the context of financing old age, are derived from their parenting practice, or their practice of being parented. In other words, they come from people's understandings of what is good for their adult children for example, on the basis of their experience of having parented them, rather than from views about the nature of property *per se*. In a very real sense, this suggests that people's inheritance practices are relationally, not materially, driven, even though the spread of home ownership means that considerations about what to do with property are becoming a more commonplace currency of English kinship negotiations.

Family property?

Our analysis of the 'case study' of financing old age has enabled us to identify some significant elements in how people reason about and use material property, and these in turn tell us a good deal about questions of ownership and kinship. We now return to these questions at a more general level, as we posed them in the introduction to this chapter, and in Chapter 1, using the concept of 'family property'. Does this have any meaning in the contemporary English context and, if not, at what points and in what ways do ideas about ownership depart from this notion?

We noted in Chapter 3 that a version of the concept of family property does seem to work for surviving spouses, where there is a clear expectation that all property will pass automatically to the other when one partner dies. However, we have argued that people do not seem to regard that process as 'inheritance', restricting their understanding of what inheritance is really about to transmission down the generations. In downward transmission, as we have argued, a 'strong' meaning of family property would be that any given generation holds ownership of property 'in trust' for the next. The property itself belongs to a transgenerational family rather than to the individual. The data from our case study of financing old age support the argument that English families have a weak sense of family property. We shall now consider this more broadly, analysing key dimensions in the concept of family property in turn and drawing in other data from our study. We shall argue that each dimension displays either weak or non-existent versions of the idea of family property.

The first dimension involves the issue of *preservation of property*. In a strong concept of family property, we would expect to see the preservation of property itself – a particular house, or piece of land, or items of furniture – across generations. There are limited ways in which such preservation of property might be achieved in English law, including the use of trusts and life interests, and the identification of specific items of property in wills.

However, there is little evidence in our sample of wills that people were thinking about property as something that should be preserved. Indeed, there is very little sense that the process of transmission is about the property itself. Only 7 per cent of wills created a trust for the whole or part of the estate. Most of these were cases involving houses where the testator's spouse is the liferent and the property reverts to the testator's children on the spouse's death. We think that this is a means of ensuring that the spouse retains the right to live in the shared home, but that the children inherit the *value* of the home on their parent's death. Our interview data, discussed below, suggest that this is not about the preservation of property *per se*, because 52 per cent of wills bequeath the estate as a single entity, without identifying any specific items as bequests ('total estate' wills). Where specific items are identified as bequests, it is normally small personal possessions like a piece of jewellery or a household ornament. Only 11 per cent of wills specified a house as a bequest, although many more of the estates in our sample must have contained one as part of the total estate or residue. The fact that major items of valuable property are not mentioned explicitly suggests that most people are not focusing on their property as such, as something whose future they wish to secure.

That conclusion would be very much supported by our interview data. In relation to the transmission of housing, there is no sense at all that people are thinking about what will happen to the house *per se* across the large number of specific comments we have about inheritance where a house is a component. The only exceptions to this are where the house is seen as providing a continuing home for people who live with the testator, normally children – as, for example, in the following extracts:

> If I died, I would like them all to live here together, Mark [her cohabitee] and the children. Then if anything happened to him, or if he remarried, the house could be sold and divided between the children.
> (Angela Sale, late 20s, divorced, home owner)

> I often think, you know, if anything happened to me and Ken got married again, this house is for the boys. What is here is for the boys, not for another partner.
> (Shirley Scott-Parker, 40s, married, first-generation home owner)

However, the point here is not so much that the children have the right to live in a particular house in perpetuity than that they are being provided for until they are old enough to set up their own home. This is an important distinction, picking up a strand that runs through our data. In the context of late twentieth-century Britain, 'a home' is a very personal creation, something that each generation expects to construct for itself and that is an important expression of individuality. Therefore, there is strong resistance to the idea of passing on 'a home' from one generation to the next, in the sense that the younger generation would occupy a home which was not of their own creation, into adult life (Finch and Hayes 1994).

Thus our data suggest that people do not think about the transmission of a house as such, certainly not as something to be preserved intact for posterity. The assumption is that, where a house is included as part of an estate, beneficiaries would want to sell it and realise its value. All of the discussions of the benefits or otherwise of equity release schemes in our case study of financing old age make that assumption. Often that would be a practical necessity, since more than one beneficiary inherits and the principle of equality in division of property requires that a house be converted into its monetary value in order to be distributed. Many of our interviewees gave us illustrations of this assumption within their own families: in Chapter 3 we quoted one example from Souresh Khan, who felt that his various properties would have to be sold and converted into money in order to ensure that his sons received exactly equal shares. A wide range of interviewees from all backgrounds take the same approach. It is clear that, in making the assumption that children normally inherit their parents' major assets, we are assuming that children inherit the value of the house, not the house itself.

We draw the conclusion from these data that there is very little sense of the preservation of property in the case of houses. Personal items are another matter, to which we return in Chapter 6. But in the case of house property – the major asset that most of the population has to bequeath – there is no sense of the importance of preserving the property as such because it is some kind of embodiment of the family. That view may well be present among aristocratic families who own properties of particular distinction or history, but for the 'ordinary' English families whom we were studying, whose property varied from modest to rather valuable, there is no apparent family attachment to the house itself. Indeed, if anything the reverse is true, since there is an antipathy to the idea that adult children could live in the 'home' created by their parents. On this criterion of how one would recognise a 'strong' view of family property, there is no evidence that it is present in the way in which contemporary English families handle inheritance.

Another criterion for recognising a strong concept of family property is that people operate on the assumption that *one generation holds property in trust for the next*, and this is the one that our case study of financing old age confronted most directly. Reviewing our data more generally, there is no evidence to suggest that property is held in trust for succeeding generations, or on behalf of preceding generations. This point has emerged strongly from our discussion of financing old age, and also from our case study of separation, divorce and remarriage (see Chapter 2). Our evidence suggests that property is not seen to be 'transgenerationally' owned or generally traceable to an ancestor.

For the most part, property is considered to be individually or jointly owned in the here and now, rather than being owned at any point in time only on behalf of an ancestral and transgenerational family, with each generation having the responsibility of passing it on to the next. Our case study of financing old age demonstrated a strong view that money and assets are *personal*. More generally, our data show that the people in our study, for the most part, do not think of the origins of assets in ancestral terms, or of ownership in transgenerational terms, even when they themselves have had some experience of inheriting from ascendant generations. There is no common concept of lineage or an ancestral 'blood line' over several generations as a route for the transmission of property, with the exception in some cases of items of personal property, which we discuss in Chapter 6. As far as major assets are concerned, we have only three examples in our data of the significance of a blood line over several preceding generations, and each is a 'weak' example of the idea of transgenerational ownership in some respect. The first is from Roy Hilton, who tells us that he sees inheritance explicitly as a matter of assets passing from father to son. He sees this system of transmission as a distinctive feature of his own family history. He is the only person in our study population who conceives of inheritance in that way. He is in his late forties and in a first-time marriage. His claims about the male line are elaborated to a considerable extent in his interview:

ROY: My side of the family have always been very careful to make sure that the money stayed in the Hiltons' hands, that it stayed in the blood line rather than going anywhere else. I

would do the same thing. There's no way it would ever go out. Straight down the line.
INTERVIEWER: Is that just the male offspring, or female as well?
ROY: Oh yes. The male.

(Roy Hilton, 40s, married, home owner)

Nevertheless, when questioned in a joint interview with his wife about their own bequeathing intentions (they have not made wills), Roy concurs with her that their estate will be divided equally between their (male and female) children. This suggests that his adherence to the principle of male descent in inheritance is likely to come unstuck in the face of the practical realities of having male and female children, and perhaps a stronger imperative to treat children equally in his own bequeathing practice. We might suggest that this is more than a little to do with philosophies of parenting as discussed above. Our other two examples involve people disapproving of, and in one case disrupting, what they see as a principle of transgenerational ownership that has operated in their families (the cases of Paul Watson and Rita Dixon, discussed in Chapter 4). There is a sense in these two cases of a rejection of what are seen as outdated and pointless practices of handing property down a blood line, and of individual generations never really owning it or having access to it.

Overall, then, our interviewees demonstrate an attachment to neither ancestry nor blood line in relation to the origins or ownership of major assets, and there is no sense at all that the people in our study see themselves as players in a historical system of transgenerational ownership. One might argue that, given that most of these families have had wealth to pass on for only one or two generations, we should expect to see this sense of commonly held property emerging in the future. Certainly, we might not expect to see a far-reaching ancestral 'gaze' in relation to property ownership from people whose families have not owned it in previous generations. We must again emphasise here that our data come from 'ordinary' families, not from those who have owned land or money for many generations. Expectations and practices there may well be different. We cannot rule out that possibility totally. However, there are other reasons to suppose that it is not just a matter of waiting for concepts of 'family' property to catch up with the experience of acquiring it. We see this by looking at the third – and slightly different – dimension of family property, and this involves following people's gaze down the generations rather than up. A strong version of family property should provide clear lines of descendancy. However, our data suggest a *limited downward generational 'gaze'* on the part of testators.

Essentially, most people are concerned with passing on to the *next* generation descendant – their children – but are not apparently greatly concerned about transmission to subsequent generations, even when they do have living grandchildren and in some cases great grandchildren. We saw this in our discussion of financing old age, and the ways in which some of those issues are tied up with philosophies of parenting (not, for example, grandparenting). The exception is families where children have divorced and married a second time, as our discussion of separation, divorce and remarriage showed (see Chapter 2). In some of these cases there is clear concern about the position of grandchildren in relation to inheritance. However, this circumstance is important precisely because it is seen as not the norm.

However, people are not normally greatly concerned about the position of their grandchildren when they talk about inheritance. The span of concern is much narrower than that. There is no evidence that John Major's vision of wealth trickling down the generations (see Chapter 1) would ever prove an inspiration for our interviewees. On the contrary, there seems to be a clear view that responsibility does not extend beyond the next generation. Grandchildren are your children's responsibility, not your own (Finch 1996). Thus there is reason to be sceptical about whether strong concepts of 'family property' and transgenerational ownership are likely to develop in future generations.

The fourth type of evidence that concepts of family property are very weak comes from the fact that *many of our interviewees believe that children do not have an automatic right to inherit*. A strong version of 'family property' should involve an expectation that children inherit from their parents. We noted the significance of this in our case study of separation, divorce and remarriage (see Chapter 2), in our discussion of inheriting money (see Chapter 4) and also in relation to financing old age, where philosophies of good parenting actually hinge on children not inheriting too much or, for some, not inheriting anything. Certainly, it is not appropriate for children to *expect* anything from their parents' estate, or to build this into their calculations and their personal economies. Furthermore, there are a few cases where an individual child has, through bad behaviour, forfeited the right to be included. Four of our interviewees, all men, talk about such circumstances explicitly.

Our fifth reason for arguing that our data show only a very weak concept of family property is the evidence that a number of our respondents demonstrate a *lack of active interest in what will happen to their own property*. In Chapter 3, we discussed the question of who makes a will and who does not and argued that even becoming a home owner with significant assets does not necessarily lead to writing a will. This in itself could be taken as an indication that many people, those who never write a will, are not interested in what will happen to their property. In reality, the situation is rather more ambiguous. Our interview data indicate that a number of people who do not write wills believe that it is unnecessary for them to do so because intestacy legislation would produce the outcome they would want in any event. Such people may be interested in what happens to their property, but only in a rather passive way, not extending to actually finding out what the law says, or what will really happen if they die intestate.

Direct evidence of lack of active interest in what will happen to one's own property comes from a group within our interview population whose comments make it pretty plain that inheritance is not a topic that has previously engaged them, beyond a passing thought. For example:

INTERVIEWER: Do you know what would happen if you died now?
MARK: No I don't. I would guess that Joanne [his cohabitee] would get half the house. I haven't really thought about it.
(Mark Lewis, 20s, single and cohabiting, home owner)

INTERVIEWER: Do you know what would happen if you both died, to your house and so on?
TOM: Not exactly, no.
INTERVIEWER: No? It's not something you've ever gone into?
TOM: No.
(Tom Brown, 40s, married, home owner)

Comments of this kind are the more striking since we told our interviewees in advance that we wanted to talk to them about how families handle inheritance issues, and therefore one might expect that this in itself would have directed individual attention to it.

Despite this, some people gave the impression that the interview itself was the first time they had thought about the subject in a personal way. Indeed, twenty-two interviewees (thirteen men and nine women) had thought so little about being a testator that it was not possible to record meaningful data on their bequeathing intentions. Given the slight predominance of women in the study population, this means that men are rather more likely than women to have given inheritance no thought. The other notable feature is that nine of this group are single and without children. However, they also tend to be among the younger interviewees and therefore the factors of marital status and age overlap. Perhaps most striking of all, nine of these people who have no meaningful bequeathing intentions are first-generation home owners, indicating that the step into owning property does not of itself lead automatically to thinking about inheritance.

We would therefore argue that, while there may be some people for whom the future disposition of their property is a matter of great importance, there are at least sizeable minorities in the population who are not particularly concerned about what is going to happen to their property after they die. This can be taken as evidence of a weak view of the transgenerational family's interest in property, the implication being that the individual has no strong obligation to secure property for his or her descendants.

Conclusion: ownership, inheritance and kinship

A clear picture has emerged in this chapter of property as generationally, not transgenerationally, owned, and notions of family property seem at best very weak in our data. More often they are non-existent.

Ownership of money and assets, especially for elderly people, is seen as inherently personal and a symbolic representation of a lifetime's labours, decisions, practices and economies, even where people have inherited part of their assets. In those cases, it seems likely that the moral practices around the use of inherited money, which we discussed in the previous chapter, help to preserve the view of money as personal against a perceived body of pressures that might treat it as a common resource. The case of financing old age helps to show that these issues of ownership are not just about whether relatives, especially children, should or should not be seen as owners in waiting. The clear answer to that is that they should not. But the issues are tied up with a changing social context in which we have witnessed not only a massive spread of home ownership but also major transformations in the role of social welfare. In particular, the role of the 'stakeholder', who should plan and organise their own welfare, and generate and accumulate assets for that purpose, has been pushed to the forefront.

In one sense, this seems entirely consistent with our analysis. The idea that elderly people can and should use their money for themselves in their old age, rather than feeling compelled to preserve it and pass it on to kin, is firmly underlined in our data. It seems a logical extension of this argument that people should engage in lifetime financial planning to cover the possible costs of care in later life, and indeed that home ownership (the accumulation of capital) is one such form of planning. On the other hand, it is against the backdrop of this move towards stakeholding, and the related changes in local government practice towards treating assets – houses in particular – as though they have been lifetime investments that can now be drawn upon to cover the costs of care, that many of people's strongest comments about the need for dignity, self-determination and choice emerge (see also Millar and Warman 1996: chapter 4). There is a firm view among most of our interviewees, young and old, that taxes should pay for care in old age, and that by the time people reach old age they will have made sufficient social and financial contributions through these mechanisms to cover the costs. The predominant view is that elderly people have already paid, and they should not be asked to pay any more. People resent the suggestion that home ownership can be seen, retrospectively, as having been a form of stakeholder planning that can now cover the costs of care. This is firmly tied up with people's understandings of what 'ownership' means – especially with the sense that it is highly personal, and that elderly people have the inalienable right to use their money and assets as they wish.

This may change over time, particularly if the notion of lifetime planning and the practice of paying for care become culturally embedded. This would mean that by the time younger cohorts reach old age they will have less of a sense than our study population appear to have that the rules have changed without their agreement. Furthermore, the strong resistance of people in our study to the idea of family property suggests that people are unlikely, *en masse*, to try to transfer assets to their children (as though they were owners in waiting) so that they can avoid paying for care, *unless* they can find ways of doing so that enable them to maintain – in their eyes and in the eyes of their kin – their own moral and personal ownership of those assets.

What have we learned about English kinship through this analysis of property 'ownership'? We began this chapter with questions about whether people use ownership of property to constitute kin relationships, and about whether and how kin relationships might influence what ownership means in the inheritance process. In some ways, our evidence – especially the absence of a concept of family property – supports Macfarlane's ideas about individualism in kinship (see Chapter 1). However, we want to suggest that much of what we have discussed actually supports the idea of relationism, more than individualism, which we also introduced in Chapter 1 and have discussed in the preceding chapters. It is clear from our analysis that people do use ownership to constitute kinship. In practices that constitute ownership as personal, generational not transgenerational, people are negotiating the appropriate balance of interdependence between kin and generations over time, in changing social contexts. It is also clear, in for example the close association between practices of good parenting and ownership in the inheritance process, that kin relationships do influence what ownership means. The processes work in both directions. Thus a picture emerges of inheritance as something that is the product of relationships or of relationism.

This is very much at odds with any idea of transgenerational ownership. For example, in a system where property is transgenerationally owned, there must be very little scope for manoeuvre and negotiation in relationships. Inheritance is necessarily governed by commonly understood rules based on genealogical position, whether or not those rules are given legal expression.

A counter argument might be that, since children do normally inherit their parents' major assets, there must be clear rules of this sort operating in practice. However, in a number of ways it is evident from our data that there are not. First, the principle of testamentary freedom itself gives legal sanction to the notion of flexibility and negotiation in inheritance. Second, and perhaps more significant, our data point to inheritance as an active and negotiated practice of kinship, not as rule-governed. This is clear in the ways in which people handle inherited money (Chapter 4) and in the often complicated processes involved in working out inheritance in 'complex' families (Chapter 2). In the case of financing old age, the strong assertion that money belongs to the person not the transgenerational family means that it can be and is being used to shape and make strong statements about kinship, and about parenting in particular.

In these ways, people's experience is not of a clear blueprint based on the idea that property belongs to the transgenerational family. Instead, their experience is of having to work out what is the best thing to do and, in the process, using inheritance to constitute their kin relationships, as well as using kinship to constitute inheritance. In the following chapter, we shall examine how inheritance of personal property fits into and extends this picture.

Chapter 6

Symbolism

Introduction: inheritance, kinship and symbolism

> The only real loss which we have had [in the family] is my Dad. Now I've got his watch – that's the only thing I can think of. It's the watch he was wearing when he died and it stopped twenty minutes after he died. So I took his watch home and I won't wind it up or anything.
> (Sheila Brent, 40s, married, first-generation home owner)

The symbolic value of personal gifts and possessions is very high and is central to people's understanding of inheritance. Sheila Brent's story of how she inherited her father's watch (a very typical personal gift) is one of many where the symbolic dimensions of inheritance are paramount. For Sheila, the watch has become a potent symbol of her deceased father because it was on his body when he died and it stopped shortly afterwards. In preserving it in that state – never winding it up and using it – Sheila preserves her father's memory through the watch.

We indicated earlier that our analysis of inheritance and kinship would consider not simply what passes to whom but the *meanings associated with objects* as they are transmitted from one owner to the next. This chapter explores that particular dimension of property transmission, which in turn allows us to examine what these symbolic dimensions of inheritance tell us about English kinship.

For this discussion of symbolism, we shift the focus to personal property because it is here that we see those symbolic dimensions of kinship and inheritance in their clearest form. By personal property typically we mean jewellery, watches, photographs or small household objects and ornaments. We have noted in earlier chapters that 'personal property' of this type appears much more prominently in the accounts of interviewees than it does in wills, where it is seldom mentioned and indeed is actively discouraged by solicitors. Typically this does not mean all personal possessions. Our data suggest that, where personal property is identified for transmission, it is *a very small number of specific items*. What is of even greater significance is the meanings people attach to property of this type when it passes through the mechanism of inheritance. We therefore focus in this chapter on personal property, its symbolic meaning, and what this tells us about family and kin relationships.

Passing on personal property: a narrative

We have chosen to approach this analysis via a construction of a narrative about passing on personal property. This narrative is a composite story, which captures the underlying themes in accounts given to us by a number of interviewees. Mostly these interviewees are talking about their own experience – of inheriting a personal item from someone else in the past, of an item they hope to inherit in the future, or one that they themselves intend to pass on. Sometimes they are talking about third parties, telling us stories about people whom they know, or friends of friends, where the point of the story is to draw out a moral or lesson. In all these accounts, we find that common themes emerge – people are talking about the same kinds of issues from similar standpoints. The basic narrative about passing on personal property goes like this:

Main narrative
   Mary is an elderly person contemplating the future of her most personal possessions.

Variation 1
1 Mary decides that the safest way to dispose of these possessions securely is to give them away while she is alive, to the precise people whom she wishes to receive them.

2   She offers them to her children or grandchildren (if she has any) or to selected others (if she does not).
3   The chosen recipient(s) may accept these gifts but feel(s) uncomfortable because these particular items symbolise Mary very strongly. It does not feel right to own them while she is still alive.
4   When Mary dies, these personal items are distributed, either according to specifications in her will (if she has one) or if there is no will, it falls to a close family member to determine how they should be distributed.

Variation 2
1   Personal items pass to children/grandchildren/others to whom Mary would have wished them to go.
2   They are cherished as 'keepsakes', as articles valued because they continue to represent Mary.
3   However, when the recipients of these objects are themselves contemplating passing on their own property, they have difficulty in working out what to do with 'Mary's keepsake' because no one in the next generation knew her personally; there is therefore some doubt about whether their meaning as 'Mary's keepsake' will be retained.

Variation 3
1   Various unscrupulous relatives manage to gain control over Mary's property and remove these special personal items along with other things.
2   The people to whom they should really have passed do not get ownership of them.
3   Thus their personal status is in some way diminished. The objects lose their meaning because the people who now own them do not value them as 'Mary's keepsake'.

This narrative contains various messages of importance to an understanding of the nature of both inheritance and kinship. Those messages centre on the concept of a 'keepsake', a word used by some of our interviewees. For example, Betty Hill speaks about having 'just a few keepsakes' from her parents, and Catherine Walmsley distinguishes 'keepsakes of remembrance' from other types of property inherited. Others use slightly different language to mean essentially the same thing: objects 'of sentimental value', 'a little reminder'. We have chosen to use the word 'keepsake' in our analysis to refer to the common idea that these different phrases express.

References to this narrative, with its different variations, occur in the accounts of fifty interviewees, about half our total. Sixteen of them simply refer to the passing on of keepsakes in a general way; the remaining thirty-four provide accounts that can be categorised as one of the variations in our narrative. Some people provide accounts of more than one such situation. Most of these accounts refer to the interviewee's own direct personal experience rather than to the reported experience of third parties.

This suggests that, in our study population, significant numbers of people are attuned to the idea of keepsakes and can talk about how they work within their own experience. Interviewees thus attuned are spread throughout all age groups, although the over-sixties are somewhat more likely than younger people to have talked to us about keepsakes. There is also a significant gender difference. About two-thirds of our women interviewees talk about keepsakes but only about one-third of men.

Central to the concept of a keepsake is the implication that an object *carries the memory* of the person who owned it but has now died. This gives the object both its meaning and its value. Its monetary value is unimportant. Indeed, the concept of a keepsake implies that the object itself is not expected to be valuable (people will refer to 'just a few' keepsakes, or an object having 'only sentimental value'). The most common types of object thus identified are jewellery (rings, watches, bracelets), with household objects or ornaments accounting for most of the rest. The emphasis is not so much on the object itself but rather on the *origin* of the object and its association with the person who owned it.

Keepsakes are therefore not 'sacred' objects in any religious sense; nor are special qualities or mystical powers attributed to the objects themselves. But they do have a special status as objects that not only symbolise but also represent a person who has died. They are therefore quite close to what Weiner (1992) has described as 'inalienable possessions', representing the kin group across generations and therefore over time.

In representing the person who has died, the keepsake acts as the *embodiment* of a person who no longer has a physical body. However, there seem to be two key requirements in order for an object to hold this status; first, that the person who now owns the object had direct knowledge of the person whose memory the object carries; and, second, that the new owner maintains an active association between the object and the person. Thus for an object to work as a keepsake requires the *active co-operation* of the person who now owns it.

In essence, these seem to be the core messages of the narrative about passing on items of personal property. We shall develop each of these further as we delve into our very rich data on this topic. We begin with the storyline of the narrative and its different variants. The concept of a keepsake makes sense of each element in the story. We have told this story from the perspective of an elderly person contemplating his or her own death, although it could be told from other standpoints. For an elderly person contemplating her or his own death, the key issue is: *how can I ensure that my memory is preserved after I die? How can I ensure that the objects most personal to me become carriers of my memory?*

This is a matter of great importance, not least to some elderly people but to some younger people as well. Much of the concern is focused upon making sure that *the right people* take possession of suitable items, so that they will become keepsakes. In most cases, it is assumed that a selected child or grandchild will be the right person, but that not every child or grandchild would be suitable. This is apparent, for example, in the following extract from Richard Murray, who talks about items that are 'too detailed' to put in a will and gives as an example an ornament of a bicycle. In talking this through with the interviewer, one can sense that he is mentally trawling through his three children to decide who would be the most appropriate recipient, rejecting one (on the grounds that she might sell the object) and deciding that others are suitable contenders (defined by Richard as 'someone with sufficient interest to keep them').

RICHARD: When you have moved on you would like to think that things have been divided up fairly and links with the past – I would like to feel that they are being retained somewhere. I mean that bicycle thing, I don't feel that some members of the family who think it's just worth selling to a second-hand shop ...
INTERVIEWER: You would want to guard against that?
RICHARD: Yes. I suppose I should see who has got the most interest. For these 'too detailed' things I would want to know that they have gone to someone with sufficient interest to keep

them, to pass them down. So I would have to discuss it between the two contenders, which would be my younger daughter and the eldest son.

INTERVIEWER: You wouldn't consider giving it to your older daughter then?

RICHARD: No, no.

(Richard Murray, 50s, second marriage, home owner)

As Richard says, the whole point about these objects going to the right person is that they would represent 'links with the past' after he has died, and he 'would like to feel that they are being retained somewhere'. He is aiming for Variation 2 of our composite narrative, the one that has the 'happy ending'. This is the most common version of the narrative as told by our interviewees. Our data contain many examples of objects successfully being turned into keepsakes after a person has died.

The following are some extracts that illustrate the range of narrative themes in Variation 2.

> I've got a Bible, well no, a Prayer Book, very small. It was given to my Dad in the trenches in the 1914 war. I'm saving it to give to [daughter's] eldest lad. Because it's a nice keepsake. And there's a nice thing on the front which tells you that it was given to my Dada, with his name, during the 1914–18 war. And that really resulted in his death, because he got a whiff of gas – but they wouldn't admit this.
>
> (Ellen Beech, 60s, married, home owner)

> When I die I'd like my best friend to have something, because we've been real good friends. I'd like her to have something of mine.
>
> (Betty Hill, 50s, widowed, council rented accommodation)

> The only thing that my father had was his watch and chain, which my eldest brother got. He's passed it on to his eldest son. So that's stayed in the family.
>
> (Toby Wallace, 60s, single, home owner)

Although it is important to many people – like Richard Murray and Betty Hill – that 'the right people' receive their most personal possessions, only a minority of keepsakes are passed on through the mechanism of a will, where the donor's intention that the recipient should have the object in question is clearly and formally stated. Partly, of course, this is because many people do not make wills, but also, where they do, we know from our solicitors' interviews and our wills data set as well as from our interviews that professionals discourage potential testators from leaving items of personal property to named individuals in their wills.

In most cases, keepsakes are indeed transmitted less formally, and we have many examples where it is simply 'understood' that a certain keepsake will go to a certain individual, because of the ways in which relationships in the family have been played out and negotiated over the years, and sometimes because of agreements reached prior to the donor's death. However, in other cases, beneficiaries of whole or part estates find themselves in a position where they have to make decisions about what items of personal property to retain, what to pass to others and what to dispose of. In doing so, they may be trying to negotiate their way through the sensibilities of many kin members and friends, and their many and varied relationships with the person who has died. They may also be trying to interpret the wishes and priorities of that person – while other kin members may be producing their own interpretations – and to uncover and adjudicate in any prior agreements about keepsakes that may have been reached between specific individuals. As a consequence, many keepsakes do come via intermediaries like a parent (who may be the son, daughter, husband or wife of the deceased, for example). On the other hand, it is not uncommon for people to select their own keepsakes from the deceased's household effects. Choosing one's own keepsake can be a highly symbolic act, but the task can also be both difficult and disputed. The informal nature of the process in many cases means that the risk of a keepsake 'getting into the wrong hands' can be great, as we shall see in our later discussion. The process of turning objects into keepsakes is therefore, for the most part, a highly interpretative activity.

Treasuring keepsakes

Although happy endings are the dominant theme of our narratives concerning keepsakes, they are not guaranteed. They have to be worked at not only by the donor but also, more importantly, by the recipient. As we have suggested, the successful conversion of an object into a keepsake requires the *active co-operation* of the recipient in maintaining an association between the object and the person, and this co-operation is most actively required once the donor is no longer around to request or oversee it. Our data suggest that people make objects they have inherited into keepsakes by 'treasuring' or 'cherishing' them, which involves a great deal more than 'just keeping' them. Many people actually use the word 'treasuring' to characterise *the way* they keep objects they have inherited. Others describe keeping items somewhere close to themselves, using or wearing them, 'never parting' with them, or keeping them on display in a central place in their homes. A few people told us that they did not particularly like the objects in themselves, but they nevertheless treasured them as a keepsake of the person who had died.

We have fifty-four examples of people keeping inherited objects (most of these are recipients' own accounts, and some give more than one example), and out of these, forty examples (given by twenty-eight individuals) are clear cases of 'treasuring' things. In these examples, the recipient is using an object as the *carrier of the memory* of someone close who has died, and of their own relationship with that person. Most of these examples concern the direct line of descent (parent–child–grandchild relationships), although some people also see this as a way of marking out a special relationship with, say, a particular niece or nephew, or a particular friend. Twenty-six of the examples of treasuring are from women (seventeen individuals) who have received keepsakes, and fourteen are from men (eleven individuals). Twenty-six of the donors are female, compared with eleven male (three were identified only as 'parents') underlining the gender difference we have already noted in the transmission of keepsakes in our data set.

Here are some examples of people talking about treasuring keepsakes:

> I've got this ornament – a pair of pot clogs – which I've always treasured. I don't think they are worth anything. It's just that I remember grandma with these pot clogs. They were in the farming community and these clogs always seemed to mean a lot to her. I don't know if they are worth anything. It's just the sentimental value. It's grandma.
>
> (Jill Pettifer, 40s, divorced, home owner)

When I think about all the baking it's done and all the foreheads it's stroked.

    (Jean Seddon, 40s, married, home owner; regarding her mother's wedding ring, which Jeans always wears)

INTERVIEWER: Did you keep anything of your auntie's?

TED: One little souvenir (gets up to get a small ornament from the top of the television – a small pottery basket about 3 inches square with a little boy inside). What it is I don't know.

INTERVIEWER: Is that something that you'd always liked when you used to visit her?

TED: Well, I remember seeing that when I was about three or four. I mean it's unusual, I mean it …

INTERVIEWER: Yeah, it's lovely. And you always keep it here in your front room?

TED: Yeah.

INTERVIEWER: Did you, you didn't take anything else of hers?

TED: No, um, I didn't want anything else.

    (Ted Beech, 70s, married, home owner)

KATHLEEN: I've got a dictionary that she [mother] won, and her brother also, one of her brothers he, um, won quite a lot of books for prizes, I can't remember now what they were for, you know, the subjects. I've got a very nice, er, lace table cloth that I was left by, by a close friend of mine, and um, you know, a vase that I've got belonged to a friend of mine that died. Her husband gave it to me, but um, memories are the things that you know, you can't see them can you?

INTERVIEWER: No, but an item could bring back the memories, is that what you mean?

KATHLEEN: Yes, or a song, and I've got records which, I went out with the boy, I was engaged to when he died, now his parents, and I've got his signet ring, and … it was after he died, some time after it, that I met my husband, but I used to wear his ring you see, I had it made …

INTERVIEWER: Smaller?

KATHLEEN: Yes, but I don't wear it now because, well, I don't think it's fair to my husband.

INTERVIEWER: No, but have you still kept it?

KATHLEEN: Oh yes, and records that his mum bought, because obviously when he died she was devastated.

(Kathleen Gregg, 50s, married, home owner)

By treasuring objects, the recipients imbue them with a range of symbolic meanings. In addition to representing the person who has died in a non-physical form ('It's grandma', says Jill Pettifer of a pottery ornament), they celebrate pride in past achievements of close kin, they underline continuity across generations, and they make statements of affection that might be less easy to put into words. Treasuring keepsakes involves keeping them in special ways and in special places, and it also involves thinking about them and talking about them in ways that are symbolic of the donor, and often very specifically the recipient's *relationship* with the donor. This comes across in a number of the extracts above and perhaps most clearly in Kathleen Gregg's feeling that to continue to wear the signet ring of the boy to whom she was engaged forty years ago would be unfair to her husband.

There are two other important points about the act of treasuring keepsakes. The first is that most of our respondents who treasured keepsakes felt the need to demonstrate that their reasons for keeping the objects, or choosing them, were nothing to do with hoarding or their own material gain, or in some cases even to do with the aesthetic or other quality of the objects themselves. People commonly say that the objects 'are not worth anything', or they go even further, as does Jill Pettifer, by saying that that they do not even know their material value – by implication, that they have not attempted to find out because owning a keepsake is absolutely not about materialism. Again, it is common for people to refer to the objects they treasure as 'small', or as having no material purpose or use. Ted Beech's account above demonstrates how an etiquette of keepsakes can operate in such a way that people may feel unable to say that they even *like* a keepsake that they have chosen for themselves, let alone that they have coveted it ('it's unusual', says Ted), because the point of the choice has to do with symbolising the person who has died and has nothing to do with personal gain. So you do not have to like an object to regard it as a keepsake and, for some people, there seems almost to be an inverse relationship between these two elements.

The final point is that treasuring a keepsake is an ongoing activity, not a once-and-for-all act. The co-operation that is required from the current owner of a keepsake is continuous and is manifested in how people continue to use and keep keepsakes, how they feel about them, and how they talk about them over time, not just on receipt of them. This means that the symbolic status of objects as keepsakes is both contingent and in need of continued reaffirmation by the current owner. If that person withdraws their co-operation at any time, potentially the status of the object as a keepsake is lost.

Keeping heirlooms

What happens in those cases where people keep objects they have inherited but do not treat them as keepsakes? Out of our fifty-four examples of people keeping things, fourteen look more like examples of 'just keeping' than of treasuring. The recipients in these cases do not feel able or willing to dispose of the objects, but they express ambiguity and sometimes some angst about what to do with them – sometimes viewing them as a burden. There is also a greater tendency to 'stick [them] in the back of a drawer' (Mark Lewis) or 'on top of the wardrobe' (Jean Seddon). What is lacking, in these cases, is a strong sense that the objects are imbued with personal symbolic significance, or that they are being used as a carrier of someone's memory. However, there is no great distinction between the types of object people 'treasure' and 'just keep'. The difference is in the way they are kept, and thought and talked about.

The word that some interviewees use to refer to objects that they have inherited but that do not have any personal symbolic significance is 'heirlooms'. We think that the concept of heirlooms is useful to describe what personal property becomes if it is inherited without being used as a keepsake. The following extract from Jane Clark's interview illustrates neatly what heirlooms are, and what problems they pose:

> I've seen my grandmother's will. I remember seeing it when I was still living at home, when I was about fifteen. She's left a sum of money to each of her grandchildren and she's got a lot of jewellery and antique things so she's just divided them out among us. She's left me quite a lot of jewellery and antique things. But I guess my Mum would probably kill me if I thought of selling them, so they'll probably just sit in the

cabinet and look pretty for the rest of their lives. She's left me a mink coat. I can't imagine what I would ever do with it. It's worth over a thousand pounds. It's really things that are family heirlooms so you can't do anything other than keep them really.

(Jane Clark, 20s, married, home owner)

Jane is clearly going to inherit quite a number of her grandmother's personal possessions, but she regards this as a burden rather than as an opportunity to embody her grandmother's memory. It is clear that the course of action that people fear – selling them – has passed through her mind and been rejected, principally because of sanctions that this would incur from her mother, who presumably has a stronger sense of objects as keepsakes. So Jane will hold on to them. They will not be lost from the family. They will assume the status of 'family heirlooms, [which] you can't do anything other than keep'. But they will have no further meaning. They will be useless objects that just take up space ('they'll probably just sit in the cabinet and look pretty for the rest of their lives'). They will be *heirlooms* not *keepsakes*.

Here are some further examples where people appear to be 'just keeping' inherited items:

My brother he inherited quite a lot of stuff from his wife's mother when she died, a lot of antiques, antique stuff. Now I think as it happens they've kept most of what was left to them. It's all in drawers and it's all shoved away in corners, but I don't think it's kept for sentimental reasons. I think it's kept more because they just don't know what to do with it.

(Tony Lewis, 40s, married, first-generation home owner)

I've got some pearls [from mother-in-law] but I don't wear them. I've got the wedding ring, her watch, but I don't, Ron [husband] said 'you can wear them' but I don't. We've got it there, sort of thing. I suppose we could give it to her granddaughter really, I suppose, eventually.

(Elizabeth Osborne, 40s, remarried, home owner)

I never wear that sovereign bracelet of his mum [her mother-in-law], and I always said to Joe, 'it's a waste of time me having this bracelet because I never wear it and all it is it's put away all the time' and I once said to the lad, David [one of her sons], 'I think I'll sell this and get a ring, something that I would wear, but he wouldn't let me sell it, David. I think he once said he'd like it if he ever got married to give to his wife, you know what I mean, but with having two children, it's a bit awkward isn't it? So I didn't know what to do about that. Still got it, I don't know what to do.

(Catherine Walmsley, 50s, married, home owner)

Why are the objects in these examples 'just kept' rather than cherished or treasured? The most obvious explanation is that the relationships in question are not as special as in our examples of keepsakes being treasured, and that may certainly explain some of these cases. The recipients simply do not see their ownership of the objects as an opportunity to embody or carry the memory of the person who has died in the rather personal and symbolic way that people who treasure keepsakes do, because the relationship between donor and beneficiary was not particularly significant to the latter.

However, we think it is significant that the main discernible differences between the composition of the group of interviewees who treasure keepsakes and those who keep heirlooms are, first, that there are no non-kin figures in the 'heirlooms' group, and, second, that our three examples involving in-law relationships fall into the 'heirlooms' not the 'keepsakes' group. There is a similar preponderance of women in both groups. The numbers here are very small and are not derived from a representative sample, so we must be cautious in how we interpret this combination of respondent characteristics and behaviour. However, it is interesting that none of our respondents felt a duty or responsibility to keep (but not treasure) objects given to them by non-kin (although some did keep *and* treasure such objects).

What does this tell us about why people actually keep objects that they do not treasure, rather than dispose of them? A consistent theme in all our examples of 'just keeping' objects is that people feel some kind of duty or imperative to hold on to them – this is how they become heirlooms rather than objects that simply disappear off the scene. Our data suggest that the concept of an heirloom as something kept but not treasured is rather specific to family and kin groups. Friendships do not generate a similar imperative, although they may form a basis for the transmission of keepsakes. In part, the centrality of kin groups here may be because other people within your family or kin group may expect you to keep such objects, even though there is little or no personal significance for you in them, and all three of our examples of gifts from parents-in-law do fit into this interpretation. In each of these cases, our respondent told us that their spouse and, in Catherine Walmsley's case her son too, would not approve if they were to dispose of the item. For Catherine, this raises complex problems because she does not want the bracelet, and she cannot sell it, but neither can she devise an equitable way of passing it on without, in her words, 'splitting it' between her sons – something she cannot do while also keeping the bracelet intact. In both of our mother-in-law to daughter-in-law examples of gifts of jewellery that have become heirlooms not keepsakes, one gets the sense that the 'real' beneficiary was probably intended to be the son/husband, but that the gift was given to the daughter-in-law/wife because it was jewellery and because she might use or wear it. But this means that the objects failed as keepsakes, because the transmission actually missed the point of keepsakes – to embody the memory of the donor under the care of a new owner who had a close enough relationship with the donor to be motivated to co-operate in this way.

As well as relationships that simply are not special enough to motivate the new owner to regard the object as a keepsake, there is the matter of relationships that are more distant over time and space. Specifically, in some of these cases the recipient's personal memory of the donor is very distant, or even non-existent. This leads us to ask: how long after someone has died can a keepsake persist? Are keepsakes possible once the personal memory of the donor has been lost?

Passing keepsakes on: from keepsakes to heirlooms?

The potential for keeping the owner's memory alive is the drive behind the creation of keepsakes; the loss of memory is the price paid for failing to achieve this. However, even if a keepsake is successfully created and cherished by its recipient, there is a question of *how long* that embodiment will last. This brings us to the question of a *second transmission* – the sting in the tale of Variation 2 of the composite narrative outlined earlier. We have already noted that direct personal knowledge of the owner is part of selecting a person as a suitable recipient of a keepsake. The converse is also true: without personal knowledge the status of the keepsake is called into question. Thus we find people who are the owners of keepsakes of their own parents will think very carefully about what should happen to this object after their own death. The following extract from Jean Seddon's interview illustrates this. Jean shows that she has thought about which of her own children would be the appropriate person to keep her own mother's wedding ring.

INTERVIEWER: [You said that you would leave] your mother's ring to [your daughter]?
JEAN: Oh definitely.
INTERVIEWER: Why? To keep it in the family?
JEAN: Yes. Well, I think she would like it because she and Mum were very close although she was only little.
(Jean Seddon, 40s, married, first-generation home owner)

In this instance, in selecting a suitable person for the second transmission of her mother's ring, Jean chooses a particular child who was 'very close' to the person whose keepsake it is. Thus the factor of direct personal knowledge, plus the likely motivation to retain the object as a keepsake, means that its status may be retained in a second transmission.

We find that the same kinds of consideration, of direct personal knowledge and likely motivation, apply in the eighteen examples we have where people pass keepsakes on to others straight away instead of keeping them themselves, or do so after some time has elapsed (but before their own death). In fact, in most of these cases we would argue that people are attempting to *preserve* a keepsake rather than to dispose of it. Most people do this where they have inherited a whole estate, or several items, and they see it as their role to distribute some of these to other kin. In other cases, for one reason or another, people feel that they have received the 'wrong' item in the original division of property and effectively swap it with someone else, usually a sibling. In most of these examples, people talk about their concern to select a suitable recipient – someone who is responsible (sometimes this is linked to reaching an age of reasonable maturity) and who will look after the keepsake. Sometimes this is linked to gender, with women being seen as more likely to 'take care of things'. The original donor in these examples is most commonly a parent, but examples also include grandparents, aunts, spouses and friends. The final recipients are most commonly the beneficiary's own children, followed by siblings, grandchildren and other kin. Interestingly, we have two examples where people who had inherited keepsakes from a friend have, after a period of years, passed them on to relatives of the original testator. Here, presumably, the criteria of direct personal knowledge and motivation to keep the keepsakes are more likely to be met than if the beneficiary had passed the objects on to his or her own kin.

In a sense, passing keepsakes on to others in this way is a way of trying to ensure that they retain their character as keepsakes, because ideally a second beneficiary is identified and the second transmission made while the memory of the original donor is still alive. By carefully choosing a second beneficiary, the first is effectively trying to secure the keepsake for another generation. It must be emphasised that it is not simply a matter of protecting the object from loss. Rather, the aim is to do this in a way which also means that it remains a keepsake, a treasured carrier of the memory of its original owner. However, options that will accomplish this are often not available, especially where someone treasures a keepsake for their lifetime before passing it to someone else on their own death. Often, at that stage, there simply is no one in the second descendant generation (still less beyond that) who had that kind of direct personal relationship with the original donor.

Thus in most cases we deduce that *an object cannot normally be retained as a keepsake through more than one transmission, less so if a long time has elapsed since the death of the testator.* For the object to work as a keepsake, the memory of the person it embodies must be strong and positive for the person who currently holds it. Thus the main exception to this general rule is in cases where the recipient at second transmission did indeed know the original owner. Mostly this occurs when a possession is passing down the line of parent–child–grandchild, but because memory is so central to the concept of a keepsake, without direct personal memories the object may be retained but its meaning changes. There is a clear danger that its status as a keepsake will be lost. In the course of second and subsequent transmissions, it becomes something else.

Lifetime transmissions: 'taking it now'

Controlling the journey and status of a keepsake is clearly a tricky business. Many elderly people worry about whether their most personal possessions will indeed go to the right person and become keepsakes. The importance of ensuring this leads some people to give away these objects while they are still alive, as in Variation 1 of the narrative outlined earlier. This solution works for some people as a way of guaranteeing the desired outcome, but it is not without its own hazards, especially from the perspective of the recipient. Younger generations may find it difficult to accept the gift while the donor is still alive, a point that comes out very clearly in the following extract from Jackie Giles, who is talking about her husband Eddie and his grandmother:

> My husband's grandmother is about eighty-odd. When his Granddad died she wasn't well herself. She was struggling to keep her house nice. So she decided that she had too many ornaments and things and she was asking the family if there was anything they would like from her house. She said that she would rather we chose things, you know, while she was still alive. And everybody did. My husband came away and said 'Oh, I couldn't take anything out of my grandmother's house', he says 'I can't break up her home like that'. You know, he's a bit funny like that. And he wouldn't. The only thing he brought was a little black elephant thing, and that was broken. He said, 'I brought that because I used to play with it as a child' (laughs). I thought, 'All these lovely antique things that she has' (both laugh), and he picks an elephant'. But you know, he's funny like that.
> (Jackie Giles, under 30, married, home owner)

In this account, Eddie's grandmother is acting consistently with our composite narrative, feeling that she is moving towards the end of her own life and asking relatives to choose objects that they will remember her by. According to Jackie's account, Eddie found this very difficult. Jackie comments that 'he's funny like that', but it is clear that she understands the emotional nature of his reaction because she remembers the incident in some detail. She remembers that he said 'I can't break up her home like that'. In fact, the object he selects is broken and not therefore a contribution to further 'breaking up' her home. It is therefore of absolutely no monetary value (which Jackie rather regrets!). However, it is absolutely the right object to act as a keepsake, since Eddie remembers playing with it as a child and therefore it is *for him* very closely associated with his grandmother. Thus, by his choice of object, Eddie creatively resolves the tension between wanting to have a keepsake and not breaking up his grandmother's home.

As well as underlining our earlier point about the difficulty of selecting one's own keepsake, this whole incident emphasises the particular character of objects as keepsakes. The reason why – at least for some people – it is very difficult to accept an object of this kind while the donor is still alive is that the very nature of keepsakes is to act as an embodiment of someone who no longer has a physical presence. The object in question needs to be something they owned and cherished if it is to act as their embodiment. Potentially, it dilutes the potency of the keepsake if a recipient starts to own it while the donor is still out there existing without it. What is more, in accepting an object intended to be a keepsake, the potential death of the donor has to be confronted directly. Indeed, it may not be stretching the interpretation too much to say that the recipient feels uncomfortable because, by accepting the object, he or she is almost willing or hastening the death of the donor. This point comes through powerfully when Sandra Fisher is talking about her mother's jewellery. Not only could she not take it now, but she doesn't even want to *think about taking it* now because it almost feels as if she would have to accept the jewellery in place of her mother:

> I presume that my mother has a drawer or something in her bedroom where all these things will be, her jewellery and things like that. I don't know. I haven't asked her you see. I don't like to ask her. I don't even like to think about it. It doesn't really interest me. I'd rather have my Mum.
> (Sandra Fisher, 40s, remarried, home owner)

Keepsakes getting into the 'wrong' hands

The poignancy of these comments ('I don't like to think about it. I'd rather have my Mum') underlines the significance of the symbolism of personal possessions as well as the discomfort that can be caused by giving them away when one is still alive. This means that it is not an easy solution. However, some people will judge that it is preferable to the danger of not doing so, namely that one's most personal possessions fall into the wrong hands, as in Variation 3 of our composite narrative. This is the 'horror story' version of the story, in which objects pass to people who know or care too little for the donor to give them symbolic meaning. Thus there are no effective keepsakes of the person who has died, nothing that carries his or her memory. The active co-operation of the recipient, an essential condition for this embodiment to take place, is withheld.

Only seven interviewees tell this variation of the narrative, either as past experiences in their circle of family or friends or as something they themselves wish to avoid with their own most treasured possessions. However, the strength of feeling gives these accounts significance beyond their numbers. The predominant feelings are disappointment at not having a keepsake of someone who has been close, and fear that one's own memory will be violated after death by objects falling into the wrong hands.

> I haven't got anything. I haven't even got a photograph of my mother or my Dad. When my Dad died, after my Mum had died, I was in America. And my sister took, she saw to it all. I don't know what happened to all the photographs to tell you the truth. I never got anything. So I haven't even got a photo of my mother. I didn't get anything.
> (Catherine Walmsley, 50s, married, home owner)

> My grandmother used to have scrolls and things. But she had a brother and he never did a good day's work in his life. But with him being the only son in my mother's family he got the lot. And he sold everything, everything, because it was his right, because he was the only son – they did in those days. [For myself] I would probably give things to my eldest son. He appreciates things. You've got to think of these things when you write a will. I'd like to know that they've gone to the right place. In my mind.
> (Dorothy Ford, 40s, married, home owner)

> My daughter-in-law was brought up by her grandmother, and we all got on very well. But at one point she got – I don't know – very strange. I had left her my jewellery. I told my daughter and she was all right, she was agreeable. But

afterwards she turned so very strange that I decided I didn't want that. So then I went and wrote a codicil, so that things were changed.

(Peggy Stevenson, 70s, widowed, first-generation home owner living in private sheltered housing)

My parents should make a will. Because I don't think I would like my sister-in-law to have my mother's jewellery. I'm not being awful but I just feel – a few times I've said to my Mum, not meaning to sound awful – 'Gail is always saying how much she likes your rings'. So I say 'This is really why you should make a will, to say that all your jewellery comes to me, and all my Dad's goes to my brother'. I get on with my sister-in-law fine but I don't think I would like her to go rooting through my Mum and Dad's house when anything happens to them.

(Jackie Giles, 30s, married, home owner)

In each of the examples above, the problem – experienced or anticipated – is that the wrong person takes intimate objects, which then lose their potential as keepsakes. This happens even if the objects ended up with the wrong person by accident, or simply got lost. It can happen even if the person who now owns the object is a close family member. For example, Dorothy Ford's great uncle inherited his parents' personal property but, despite being their eldest child, he proved to be the wrong person to hold their keepsakes.

In that particular case, there was also a concern that he would dispose of these personal items altogether. This can indeed happen. We have two cases in our study population where the interviewee reports having had to 'rescue' treasured personal possessions from imminent sale. One of these is Sandra Thompson, whose father sold her mother's jewellery after the latter's death; Sandra realised this in time to buy back just one item:

When my Mum died my Dad took all her jewels – they didn't have any value at all – to the local jewellers and sold them. Which hurt me. I mean he could have said 'Wouldn't you like something special of your Mum's?' We just couldn't understand it at all. And we found out where he had sold them and I bought one of my Mum's things. It was this little cameo. I saw it in the window and it was the only thing left – the shopkeeper had sold all the rest. So I bought it back, and he let me buy it for what he had given my Dad, not the price in the window. I mean the amount of money that my Dad must have got for the jewels was quite small compared to the sort of value they would have had if he had passed them all on to the children.

(Sandra Thompson, 50s, widowed and cohabiting, home owner)

This poignant tale of insensitivity and resentment powerfully underlines what is lost when a potential keepsake is denied to the person who wants to use it as such. But even if the property is not lost for good it will still be the in 'wrong place' for a prized personal object if it ends up with a person who will not treat it as a keepsake. Thus Jackie Giles (in the extracts above) worries about her sister-in-law 'rooting through' her parents' possessions, treating them as objects to be retained or rejected on grounds of taste or value, rather than as objects that could continue to embody their owner. Similarly, Peggy Stevenson changed her will, removing the previous bequest of jewellery to her daughter-in-law, when the latter 'turned so very strange'. She made this change not because she thought that the daughter-in-law might dispose of the jewellery; she did so because she lost confidence that she would treat the jewellery as Peggy's keepsake.

Thus it is clear that the problem of special items of personal property getting into the wrong hands is that *the memory of the owner is lost*. There is no embodiment of the person after he or she has died; indeed, the deceased's most personal possessions are discarded as worthless or prized only for their monetary value. The owner's status is thereby diminished and his or her memory potentially contaminated. There is also a loss of status for the person who 'should' have received the object and who would have treated it as a keepsake. That person is denied the opportunity, which he or she would have valued, of retaining the memory of the person who has died, embodied in their most personal possessions.

Conclusion

Through our analysis of data on the transmission of personal property we are able to see that there is a clear identification between people and objects, and that the preservation of this over time – and especially after someone has died – is a key feature of inheritance. The interview data on personal property are, as we noted in Chapter 3, more extensive than for other kinds of property. People talk about it more, are more concerned to get it right, and the examples reviewed in this chapter demonstrate real emotional power. Under the right circumstances, property of this sort can clearly be both representative of the past and confirming of individual standing and relationships for the present and future. As we noted in our discussion of Weiner's work (see Chapter 1), possessions transmitted and treasured across generations can confirm individual identities, the significance of kinship over time and a sense of continuity in a changing world (Weiner 1992).

The use of objects in this way, as carriers of memory that continue in some sense to 'be' the person who has died, and to symbolise the recipient's relationship with them, is more characteristic of women than men. Nevertheless, there are a number of men – one-third of the men in our study population – who do think about objects and relationships in the same terms. A number of them are quoted above, and it is clear that the process of identifying keepsakes is as important to them as it is to many women. Conversely, it is also true that women do not inevitably think about objects and relationships in these terms, as for example in the case of Jane Clark regarding her grandmother's possessions as just useless heirlooms. A more useful line of enquiry may be to ask what it is about women's lives that may lead them to more often have formed the type of close relationships with kin that they then wish to preserve through keepsakes. We shall return to these issues in a discussion of gender in Chapter 7.

Our analysis of keepsakes also brings out the relational and personal nature of the process, on both sides. The donor selects both an object and an individual recipient and matches them together. The selection of the recipient often comes from the same range as those who receive major gifts – children and grandchildren – but not exclusively so. On the recipient's side, there must be a desire to go on actively acknowledging the importance of one's relationship with the donor after he or she has died. So, in contrast with major gifts, where the principle of division is equality between people of equivalent genealogical status, in the transmission of personal property a distinction is made between one child and another, sometimes explicitly on grounds of suitability for the role of guardian of keepsakes. All of this suggests an active and relational form of inheritance practice that constitutes kinship in highly specific ways for different individuals.

We have also uncovered an important angle on the issue of 'family property' in this analysis. The fact that our interviewees seem much more emotionally engaged with individual keepsakes (often objects of no value) than with material resources transmitted through inheritance suggests a very weak view of family property in the sense of a common state in economic resources across generations. At the same time, there is, for many of the families in our study, a clear symbolic stake in specific items of personal property that can act as keepsakes.

Chapter 7
Drawing conclusions
Kinship and inheritance

Introduction

We began this book with a set of questions about how kinship and inheritance are connected. We pointed out right at the beginning that this is a book about *kinship* more than inheritance. Our interest throughout has been in what inheritance reveals about kinship in the English context. However, we have suggested that inheritance is more than a lens on kinship. When people make decisions about whether and to whom to pass their property when they die, or what to do with something they have inherited, they are in the business of constituting kinship, not just reflecting it. Inheritance is a central feature in the *making* and *doing* of kinship and has become more so with the spread of home ownership, which makes inheritance a live issue for a much greater proportion of the population than in even the recent past.

In this chapter, we shall pull together and develop our arguments about how inheritance constitutes kinship. In the process, we also reflect on the converse: how kinship constitutes our understandings of the meaning of inheritance and the concepts of property and ownership on which it is based. We shall do this by exploring four sets of issues. First, what is kinship, and where is it located socially? Second, what is the significance of gender? Third, how do symbolism, morality and materialism interrelate in inheritance and kin relationships? Fourth, what is the significance of time?

Locating kinship

Conventionally in social science literature, kinship is referred to as a 'structure' or a 'system'. Our empirical analysis suggests that, *if* kinship is a structure or system, then it is much more consistent with an 'individualistic' one as envisaged by Macfarlane (1978) than with one based on descent within fixed genealogical positions. We argued in Chapter 1, following Macfarlane, that an individualistic kinship structure is 'ego-centred' in the sense that each individual is the centre of their own kin universe rather than joining a pre-existing ancestor-centred family. Macfarlane's analysis suggests that property ownership and transmission in ancestor-centred kinship systems is structured around the concept of lineage in two senses. First, property remains with the 'community of males', following male lines of descent; and second, property is owned by any one generation only on behalf of the lineage, a form of ownership that we have called 'transgenerational'. For Delphy and Leonard, writing about families and property in France, these concepts come together in the practice of 'patrimony', which concentrates power and privilege in the hands of eldest male heirs (Delphy and Leonard 1992).

We interrogated our own empirical data against Macfarlane's 'proofs' of ancestor-centred or lineage-based kinship in our data. We find no evidence of either. In relation to the first, property does not belong to the 'community of males' in the non-aristocratic English families that we have studied. The principle of equality in the division of major assets between children, whatever their sex or birth order, is one that people hold very dear according to our interviewees. This was supported by data from our interviews with professionals involved in wills and probate, and in the patterns of bequeathing we traced in our sample of wills. In relation to the second, as we have discussed quite fully in the preceding chapters, we can find little or no evidence for the operation of transgenerational ownership of major assets in any of our data sets, and instead we find that the idea of generational ownership is strongly asserted. There is one possible exception to this: the constitution and transmission of 'keepsakes', which we examined in the previous chapter. However, our analysis clearly indicates that this does not constitute transgenerational ownership. Far from representing a common stake in economic resources across the generations of 'a family', keepsakes celebrate and symbolise *particular relationships*, usually with items of little material value, and only for as long as the personal memory of the owner is retained.

So our analysis tells us that kinship, for inheritance purposes, is not organised around ancestry or lineage in these senses. There is no concept of 'patrimony' in the English context, nor is one emerging. However, kinship should not necessarily be seen as constituting an individualised structure. That concept does not quite seem to capture what we recognise as kinship in our own analysis, or how people tell us they experience their kin relationships. The interrogation of the concept of individualised kinship can be broken down into two questions: is English kinship a structure or a system? Is it individualised? These questions naturally lead on to wider ontological concerns about the nature of kinship, and its social or cultural location, which our data can help us to address. These are as follows: what is kinship? How is it constituted? Where does it exist or take place? And where is it done?

Clearly, the answers to these questions may be many and varied, but on the basis of our data we can offer some reasonably robust answers. First, we think that kinship operates at, or is to be found at, the level of *negotiated relationships* more than structures or systems. The body of our data points in this direction, with its emphasis on inheritance as a product and practice of relatedness and the ways in which people handle and express this. Relationships are created and sustained through contact, conversation and a common life over long periods of time – processes that elsewhere we have characterised as negotiations (Finch and Mason 1993). Some of these negotiations are about inheritance. Essentially, this is why we wish to jettison both the idea of kinship as a structure and the concept of individualism in favour of one of *relationism*.

Second, we want to suggest that kinship is constituted in *relational practices*, with the privilege that this concept gives to actors' reasoning, actions and experiences. This is how the morality and symbolism of kinship are expressed – for example, in the practices associated with using inherited money, or with treasuring keepsakes – rather than through established rules or norms about what appropriate kinship must look like. Again, we are building on our earlier work here, as well as on the use of Morgan's concept of 'family practices' (Finch and Mason 1993; Morgan 1996; Smart and Neale 1999). The scholarly search for 'rules' of kinship, or of morality, suggests and imposes too static an order on what our data tell us are complicated, fluid and active practices, forms of reasoning and ways of dealing with often conflicting issues in daily life. In this sense, kinship is very much about *doing, reasoning and working it out in your own relationships*. Where consistencies emerge in how people do these things, we do not feel that this should be interpreted to mean that underlying rules have produced them (or that they constitute a 'structure' or 'system') and hence that kinship is constituted through following rules. Consistencies are interesting, of course, and in places we have identified some common principles that people both appeal to and activate in their practices. However, we would argue that the analytical focus should remain upon the practices, not the principles, since these are the drivers, the motors, of kinship.

The meaning attributed to consistencies in kinship practices brings us to our third point: kinship is constituted in and through *narratives*. We have used the concept of narrative as a methodological and analytical device to illustrate some of the consistencies in our interview data but, more than that, to communicate accounts and scenarios that people recognise and, most notably, that they fear. In this sense, the narrative is an expression of people's attempts to connect their own experiences and reasoning to something that they perceive to be more generalised, and the significant point is that many people do this. The narratives we have used tend to be expressions of what people think should not happen, or what they do not want for their own families, and are scenarios that they actively try to avoid. This means that the stories that the narratives contain do not of themselves represent an empirical and generalisable reality of kinship. They do not describe what people generally do, nor do they represent moral rules about what they should do. However, we learn about people's practices and moral reasoning through them because many people use narratives like those we have sketched out to locate and make sense of their own (usually oppositional) practices. This means that the construction of generalising narratives as a way of contextualising their own practice is an important element in the way in which people *do* kinship and inheritance.

Third, our data strongly suggest that kinship is constituted in *sentiment and memory*, which essentially form part of the relational practices that we have already identified. Our analysis of keepsakes pointed to the importance of memory, as well as sentiments and feelings about specific relatives, in understanding how inheritance works in families, and hence we would argue that these elements are absolutely central to the meaning of kinship. We shall discuss the concept of memory more fully when we explore what our data say about the significance of time for kinship.

Finally, we need to consider how far kinship is constituted by economy or materiality. Here we draw out a major conclusion from our analysis of inheritance, and what this tells us about kinship. *We do not believe that the nature of kinship can be expressed or is constituted predominantly in material terms.* We do not wish to deny that economic resources are transacted in kin relationships. Nor do we wish to underplay the significance of inheritance, especially in the context of the spread of home ownership, for changing patterns of wealth distribution, and the part that family and kin relationships play in that process. Undoubtedly, the links between housing and family wealth are significant, and we agree that we need to understand more about them if we are to document, explain and predict changing patterns in the distribution of wealth (Forrest and Murie 1995; Franklin 1995; Munro 1987). However, our study was designed to help us to understand kinship rather than to read the significance of kinship for wealth distribution. In this context, it is one thing to say that kin relationships influence patterns of wealth but quite another to say that kinship is driven by or is principally about economic factors.

Clearly, changing economic patterns, such as the spread of home ownership, influence the nature, amount and currencies of economic resources that are transacted in kinship. The mere fact that potentially more people than before have something of economic value left when they die raises questions about what can and should be done with those resources. It is significant that in contemporary English society these seem to be seen by most people, and more ambiguously perhaps by the law and the state, as *questions for kinship*. So in the sense that changing matters of economy raise issues for kinship to deal with, we must agree that kinship is implicated in and has consequences for economic processes. We shall discuss these issues further shortly in our analysis of the relative roles of symbolism, morality and materialism in inheritance practices.

In summary, we believe that English kinship should be regarded as a set of processes or practices much more than a structure or system. It is certainly not a pre-existing structure into which individuals are slotted through accidents of birth or choices like marriage. Our study has given clear evidence that individuals expect to 'create' a family rather than to 'join' one.

It is this 'creation' of kinship that we describe as a set of processes or practices. These practices are relational, and they are active. They are made and remade over time as each of us works out our own relationships with others with whom we share ties of blood, legal contract or other commitment. This process of working out relationships necessarily entails not only 'doing' but also 'reasoning', creating one's own understandings of the meaning of the relationships in which one is involved. That reasoning can operate on different levels, but it does not necessarily entail 'rules of conduct'. Rather, we have highlighted the importance of narratives – the stories that people tell themselves and others to enable relationships to be situated and understood in a shared way.

These practices work at different ontological levels and over time. As we see it, kinship is continually being made or crafted by people in different and changing social locations, with different experiences, concerns, gazes and existences. It is important to emphasise two points here. First, we are not saying that kinship is based on infinite, individual variety. There are consistencies and common concerns. Instead, we are saying that the English context produces kinship that is both fluid and dynamic, and that this is the norm not the exception. It perhaps explains why, in the English context, kinship practices often seem to defy attempts to pin them down in legislation or social policies.

Second, nor are we arguing that the form which kinship takes is a direct consequence of people's specific social positions. Our analysis in previous chapters suggests that factors like genealogical position, age, gender, wealth, ethnicity and marital status do not function like variables that correspond to distinctive kinship practices. Indeed, in relation to ethnicity, although our numbers of non-white British interviewees were small (see Appendix A), there are more similarities than differences in inheritance practices across ethnic divisions among our interviewees.

However, people's life experiences are highly salient to their reasoning, and to the contexts in which their practices are developed. Such life experiences include those we have discussed in previous chapters: divorce, separation, repartnering and step-relationships (as discussed in Chapter 2); being the first generation in one's family to own a house (as discussed in Chapter 5); being part of a transnational kin group (as discussed in Chapter 4); or being in a position where the contemplation of one's own or a relative's death becomes a live issue (linked to age, but not determined by it, as discussed in Chapters 3, 5 and 8 (see also Finch and Wallis 1993). These life experiences tend to be relational, not individual, and therefore do not translate into individual characteristics or variables. What they do is to raise distinctive sets of issues in people's lives, and in some senses provide contexts, perspectives and changing locations. But they do not straightforwardly determine inheritance or kinship 'outcomes'.

Gender, inheritance and kinship

One dimension of experience that is relevant for inheritance and kinship is that of gender. We have commented in earlier chapters on gender differences and patterns in our data, and we want now to draw these comments together and discuss their significance. We shall focus on three broad areas, which, taken together, reinforce our general point that experiences play a more prominent role in shaping kinship than do ascribed social positions.

First, in terms of 'who gets what' in transmissions of property via inheritance, one of the most striking features of our data is that testators do not differentiate between male and female beneficiaries in relation to major assets. Sons and daughters, for example, get equal shares. Where differentiation does occur it is in personal property, with a tendency – though not an absolute rule – for gifts to be transmitted in gender-specific ways: jewellery from and to females, for example. In terms of these broad patterns, therefore, and especially in relation to the transmission of economic resources, gender does not appear to be a highly prominent feature.

Second, if we look at testators, our wills study reveals a tendency for men and women to write different types of last will (see Chapter 3). Men are more likely than women to write 'total estate' wills with their spouse as main beneficiary. Women are more likely than men to write some form of complex or 'composite' will, with a wider range of beneficiaries. We have suggested that in part this is likely to be a function of demography, where wives are more commonly the 'survivors of the married couple'. It is also a consequence of the almost universal practice of joint ownership of major assets between married couples. In situations where assets pass 'automatically' to the survivor of the couple (more often the woman) on the first death, that survivor may effectively 'control' inheritance to descendant generations, unless they repartner (Finch and Hayes 1995). This potentially gives some women a prominent position in relation to transmission of property through inheritance. It also means that women may more frequently face decisions about 'financing old age' of the kind we discussed in Chapter 5. However, we should emphasise that these patterns are not entirely clear-cut, and there are variations in the shape and form of wills written by both women and men (Finch et al. 1996).

Third, and perhaps most significantly, women appear to take a leading role in the symbolic practices associated with inheritance. In particular, we noted a greater involvement of women than men in the transmission and treasuring of keepsakes through which some kin relationships were commemorated and symbolised (see Chapter 6). Women were also more likely than men to spend inherited money in commemorative ways, or to find a symbolic connection in what looked like more mundane purchases (see Chapter 4). Again, however, we must emphasise that around one-third of the men in our study were also involved in the symbolic practices associated with keepsakes, and conversely that a significant minority of the women apparently were not. This means that symbolism in kinship is not a straightforwardly gendered practice.

The transmission and treasuring of keepsakes can nevertheless be confirming of gender identities and of moral reputations in families, and we can identify two elements in this process. First, as we noted in Chapter 6, the choice of a suitable recipient for a keepsake is for some people directly to do with gender, because 'women take better care of things'. While not everyone saw it in these terms, no one suggested that men in general 'take better care of things', even though some men had certainly been entrusted as individuals with keepsakes in their own families. Second, the selection of a 'gender-appropriate' gift for a beneficiary, although not a universal practice, is common and says something about how people perceive women's and men's relationships to particular types of object and possession. These elements come together in cases where a 'female' gift is given to a beloved daughter or niece because she will take care of it and look after the memory it symbolises. This both confirms and celebrates women's family reputations as people who are trustworthy, sensitive and attuned to the needs of others: as good relational beings who take care of things and relationships.

Many people recognise these two sets of images, whether or not they match their own lived experience of kin relationships. In that sense, the symbolic practices associated with keepsakes constitute a *gendered narrative* that helps to construct, culturally speaking, a particular kind of *female family identity*. There is not a corresponding male family identity, even though specific examples of men's involvement in transmitting and treasuring keepsakes are not uncommon.

Taken together, these data suggest that there is a tendency for men and women to have different experiences of and involvement in processes of inheritance and hence in the constitution of kinship, with women occupying a more central position in some respects. However, these differences are quite subtle and are not entirely clear-cut. There is variation within gender categories as well as between them.

We think the differences can be explained, at least in part, by material, cultural and relational realities of women's lives, which tend to give them plenty of practice in 'relationship work' (see Mason 1996a). Our earlier work on family responsibilities demonstrated that, in general, women are more firmly locked into sets of family responsibilities and more finely attuned to the sensibilities and negotiations through which they are created, although again in that study we noted considerable variation across gender categories (Finch and Mason 1993). In this sense, it is not surprising to find women taking the leading role in the active moral, relational and symbolic practices through which inheritance is organised and kinship constituted. Women are more likely to have formed the kind of close personal relationships with kin that they wish to symbolise and celebrate in some way, and they may have gained more practice in the active relational work that is involved in treasuring keepsakes, for example.

So, although our data demonstrate that there is not a *necessary* congruence between gender and inheritance practices, there are some associations, and the gendering of family identities is a key element. This is undoubtedly underscored by the tendency we have already mentioned for women to be 'the survivor of the couple' and in that sense to predominate, demographically speaking, in controlling the process of inheritance down the generations.

A consideration of the significance of gender therefore reveals a rather subtle and nuanced picture, in which the demographic, material, cultural and relational realities of women's and men's lives interweave. It also paints a picture of inheritance in which material and economic factors seem relatively unimportant when compared with the moral and symbolic practices associated with keepsakes. This raises in stark form the question to which we have said we shall return: to what extent is kinship constituted by economy or materiality? In order to answer this question, we shall throw the focus directly onto the relationship between symbolism, morality and materialism in inheritance practices.

Symbolism, morality and materialism

There are a number of key points in our overall analysis of inheritance practices that help us to examine the relationships between symbolism, morality and materialism. Perhaps the most significant is that our interviewees' accounts suggest that there is no responsibility to pass on material assets through the mechanism of inheritance, although many people do express a desire to do this if they can. Our analysis of financing old age, for example, suggested that elderly people are seen as having inalienable rights to control their own resources, and to decide whether to reserve anything to pass on as an inheritance or not. The corollary of this is that receiving an inheritance is treated as a bonus, an extra, or 'a treat' as Josie Lewis (one of our interviewees) put it. It is definitely not treated as a necessity. It is not seen as legitimate for people to calculate inheritance into their personal, or household, or routine economies. This is partly why, as we showed in Chapter 4, people find it difficult to know how to deal with inherited money. If it were part of their routine economies it would not present such a challenge. This idea of bonus rather than necessity also finds expression in the more general principle which our data support: that it is wrong to expect an inheritance.

All of these points, as we have argued, point towards the idea that material resources are generationally not transgenerationally owned and away from the notion of family property. We can take from this the basic point that kinship does not have to be underwritten by material resources in order to have meaning. Yet the picture is more complex and nuanced than that. In elaborating this basic analysis, we can identify three sets of practices in which people are engaged and that help us to explain both the consistencies and the differences that we have documented in our interview data. Each of these sets of practices provides a view of the relationship between symbolism, morality and materialism in the ways in which people 'do' kinship through inheritance. The three are looking after memories; recognising specific relationships; and good parenting. We shall discuss each in turn.

Looking after memories

In the previous chapter we argued that, in creating keepsakes, people are dealing with memories. For those contemplating their own death we argued that the key issue is how to ensure that personal objects become carriers of one's own memory. As we explained, our interviewees demonstrated that they expend much mental and emotional energy in selecting the right person for a specific object. This choice is made on the basis of the histories of particular relationships rather than on an assumption that all occupants of a 'kin position' (for example, all of one's children) would be equally suitable, although we have noted the significance of gender in the process. The point is that people try to select beneficiaries who will look after their memory appropriately by turning the object into a keepsake. Viewed from the opposite angle, when people inherit objects and turn them into keepsakes, they are looking after the memory of the donor in a very active fashion rather than simply keeping an object because they remember the person. Essentially, they are using the object to become the symbolic representation or the embodiment of their relationship with that person and, in the process, they are *animating* memory – creating, shaping and sustaining it – not just keeping it. Very often, this process involves objects with little or no material value, and it is clear that looking after memories entails showing a strong lack of interest in any material value or otherwise that an object may have. In this sense, then, looking after memories through keepsakes is an active and symbolic practice of kinship and, as we have argued, people have a very strong emotional engagement with these issues. For many people, this is what inheritance is really about.

To some extent, our interviewees engaged in these kinds of memory practice when they made decisions about how to use inherited money too. Unlike keepsakes, however, money cannot simply be kept as a symbolic representation of the donor without moral risk to the beneficiary, yet neither is it straightforwardly viewed as a part of people's routine or personal economies. Inheriting money is 'a bonus', and recipients are confronted with moral dilemmas about its use. In trying to resolve these, we showed that people again seek to honour and activate memory of their relationship with the person who has died. Making money 'special' in a range of ways is a central element in this, but sometimes this conflicts with the demands of people's routine or personal economies. This becomes manifest in difficult questions about whether the beneficiary should give priority to the memory of their relationship with the person who has died, or to their own current economic commitments. Most people strive to prioritise the former, while recognising the latter. We argued that in this sense beneficiaries are operating at the interface between a past family (the 'inheritance' family of the person who has died) and one version of a present family (the 'economic' family of the beneficiary, that is, the family among which resources are routinely shared).

The practices involved in looking after memory are, therefore, predominantly to do with working out symbolic and moral issues within sometimes complex sets of relationships. In a strong sense, these practices are relationally driven. Inheritance of money injects economic considerations into these processes, but essentially this too is dealt with in the same ways.

Recognising specific relationships

The practice of looking after memories is predominantly undertaken by people who become beneficiaries in the inheritance process, although we have also suggested that testators engage in these processes to the extent that they are concerned with the preservation of their own memory. One set of practices that is characteristic of testators more than beneficiaries, however, involves recognising specific relationships. Our analysis of keepsakes in Chapter 6 and our discussion of small cash bequests in Chapter 3 both brought to the fore the ways in which people may use the transmission of these items – usually of little material value – through inheritance to recognise the specificity of relationships, rather than a uniformity based on genealogical positions. We argued in these chapters that the range of kin (and non-kin) identified as beneficiaries of such gifts was quite wide and, more importantly, was highly variable between testators. It is very common for children to receive such gifts alongside major assets from their parents' estates. The practice of passing on personal items is widespread. It often occurs informally outside a will, and although it generally involves gifts of little economic value, as we have suggested this in some sense is what inheritance is really about for many of our interviewees.

Specificity in relationships is also consistent with the idea that testators should be able to *choose* whether and how to transmit their assets and possessions, which is so firmly underlined in our data. This is thrown into sharp focus in the context of divorce, separation, repartnering and step-relationships, discussed in Chapter 2. The main emotional bite of the narrative we presented there about property 'passing out of the family' was the dreaded possibility that property could end up in the hands of someone whom the testator would not have chosen and with whom they had no personal relationship. This overall message about what might constitute 'passing out of the family' was crucially about specificity and choice in relationships more than any fixed concepts of the 'blood line' or the preservation of family property.

Overall, then, the practices involved in recognising specific relationships, a significant element of what inheritance is about, are relationally more than materially driven.

Good parenting

Children hold a special place in the inheritance process viewed from the perspective of testators, and our conclusions about kinship must take that on board. We pointed out in Chapter 3, on the basis of all three of our data sets, that, looking across the board, beneficiaries of major assets are spouses first, then children. We also argued that people do not think that property passing to a spouse constitutes inheritance, primarily because of the assumption that married individuals hold property in common. If spouses are removed from the inheritance picture, then the dominance of children as beneficiaries of major bequests is very clear. Typically, if there is no surviving spouse, children get a share of the total estate or residue. The principle of equality is very strong indeed in relation to transmissions to children, and for most people that means strictly equal divisions irrespective of the different life circumstances of children, or of quality of relationship, birth order or gender. In a minority of cases in our interview study, exceptions to the principle of equality were made on the basis of prior economic ties between parents and one child, or clear and distinct needs or claims on the part of one child. Essentially, these were cases where special treatment was designed to achieve some form of equality of outcome, or a fair outcome. However, what is more striking is the rarity of such examples.

The distinction between equality of treatment and of outcome is one that surfaces more significantly in relation to step-children in our study, where bequests from other sets of parents are sometimes included in the testator's frame of reasoning and sometimes are not (see also Flowerdew 1999). Step-children may or may not be treated on equal terms with biological children but are more likely to be so in cases where the step-parenting relationship is established early in the child's life.

We think that the impulse to equality in the treatment of children in inheritance is best explained in relation to a wider set of practices concerning 'good parenting'. The principle of equality between children is one that other researchers have noted is paramount in parenting practice (*ibid.*), yet in many aspects of family life it is difficult or impossible to achieve. This is not least because equality, in so far as it suggests sameness, is not a good *relational* concept: one simply cannot have exactly the same relationship with different people. Research on children in families has pointed to their active role in constructing family relationships and in positioning themselves in competition with their siblings on a range of issues (see especially Brannen 1999). Parenting practice in this context becomes, in part, the art of demonstrating equal treatment and a lack of favouritism, and by the time the children reach adulthood parents may be very experienced in this. Parenting in step-families is particularly likely to produce a highly active engagement with these issues because of the more complex contexts in which it is performed (Flowerdew 1999). In a sense, then, it is probably because of the very variability and individuality of parent–child relationships, and the patterns of daily life on which they are grounded, that the impulse to equality in parenting *where it can be demonstrated* is so strong.

Inheritance of money and major assets is one domain in which equality of treatment can be demonstrated. The convention of dividing total estates into proportionate shares makes the relative size of each portion entirely visible, and the currency of money is one that is similarly transparent. Where the medium of a will is used, the transparency of the process is enhanced. We want to suggest that these mechanisms for apportioning equal shares are used to champion the principle of equality of treatment as a key element of good parenting practice. In other words, people are using inheritance, and the opportunity it provides for passing on material resources, to make strong statements about, or to construct a *narrative* of, good parenting practice rather than necessarily to direct resources in specific ways or to enhance 'family wealth'. At the same time, the passing on of specific items of personal property as keepsakes to selected individuals allows parents simultaneously to recognise specificity in their relationships with their children and others. It is a little like saying: 'I love all of you the same, but this is what is special about my relationship with you'. Money is reckoned on a single and universal scale. Objects are not. And, of course, children have a whole range of possibilities for looking after their parents' memories in ways that can symbolise the specificity of their relationship with that parent.

Practices of good parenting also help to explain different perspectives, reflected in our data, on the issue of whether or not parents have a clear responsibility to pass anything on to children through inheritance. Should a parent ensure that he or she holds back enough savings or assets to guarantee that there will be something for the children after she or he dies?

As we argued in Chapter 5, for the most part this issue is seen in terms of choice, not responsibility, and the message that elderly people have the right to use their money as they choose is very strong. Different philosophies of what constitutes good parenting can be used to support the practice of passing on 'something', or of not passing on anything at all, or at least not 'too much'. What underpins these appeals to good parenting is the concept of independence between generations and, specifically, the responsibility of the older generation for fostering and facilitating the independence of the next, either by giving them a 'good start' or by helping them to learn to fend for themselves. It is this relational matter, not a responsibility to pass on material resources and certainly not a notion of transgenerational ownership of resources, that explains people's inheritance practices.

The three sets of practices – looking after memories, recognising specificity and good parenting – clearly interweave material, moral and symbolic dimensions in the inheritance experience. However, none of them is primarily or even predominantly about materialism. We would argue that in each area people's practices are relationally driven, and relationally grounded. Material elements get used in these processes, but in no sense can we conclude, on the basis of our study of inheritance, that kinship is sustained by or is constituted in predominantly material terms.

Inheritance, kinship and time

Our picture of inheritance is one that has people working out how to construct and pursue relationships over time. It is both complex and fluid and, as we have suggested, it is not really an 'it' at all. Indeed, if we examine the shape of the family or kinship that is constituted through these various practices, in the sense of which kin are included and excluded, we get a range of different versions. There is not a static or singular picture of 'the family' that emerges.

There are two main explanations for this. The first is that inheritance is constituted in practices (for example of memory, selection, parenting) that a whole range of people may be undertaking in relation to others, and each will be constituting *different versions* of 'my family'. So, for example, the woman who is deliberating about who should have her most personal possessions is highly likely to select a range of kin (and perhaps non-kin) based on the quality and history of her relationships with them rather than on any formal set of rules for reckoning genealogical closeness. At the same time, she may have made the assumption that her major assets will be passed to her husband, or divided equally between her children, on the basis of either the logic of shared ownership between spouses or a philosophy of good parenting. The nephew who receives one of her personal possessions and turns it into a keepsake will in so doing activate a memory of his relationship with her, which is not the same as the woman's full range of family relationships as she would have envisioned them. The daughter who receives a half share of her major assets may similarly activate her personal/relational memory of her mother in the ways she chooses to spend or invest the money, but she will also be negotiating with a version of her own family based on her routine domestic economy. This rather limited 'domestic economy' version of family is unlikely to match what that same daughter would construct as her 'inheritance family' when thinking about the transmission of her own assets and personal possessions. And so on.

The more general point here is that people's version of 'my family' is constituted through different sets of practices at any one time, and there may be different versions of 'my family' at any given time. The different versions intersect at various times, through the relational practices of people, as in our scenario that has a daughter at the interface between her mother's 'inheritance family' and her own 'domestic economy family'. This is what any bigger picture of what kinship is has to take on board.

This leads to our second explanation for the complexity and fluidity of kinship. This centres on concepts of *time and perspective* through which practices like looking after memory, recognising specificity and good parenting are constituted. Some of the differences in the versions of family outlined above are due to the differential locations of the actors involved in concepts of family time and, in particular, whether their current preoccupation is 'looking down', generationally speaking, 'looking up' or 'looking across'. It is not so much that these gazes provide different perspectives on the same thing but that they constitute that 'thing'. In her analysis of time and social theory, Adam has argued that

> All human action ... is embedded in a continuity of past, present and future, extends into the past and future; and constitutes those horizons whilst binding them in a present.
> (1990: 127)

In a sense, inheritance does this *par excellence*. It has a special place in the constitution of families and kinship over time. To put it another way, inheritance practices constitute *kinship as a way of organising time*. Inheritance positions people at the interface between different versions of family: both their own and other people's, but also those located in past, present and future, and it ties these 'horizons' into the present. The past, the present, the future can be perceived in terms of these intersections of different versions of 'my family'.

However, what is perhaps rather striking, especially in a study that potentially foregrounds the transgenerational possibilities of kinship, is the limited temporal span that even the intersections of different versions of 'my family' produce. We have argued that people, when 'looking up' generationally speaking, do not have an ancestral view and instead usually look after the memory of only selected people from one prior generation. The element of specificity in that process also limits the breadth of that antecedent view. When 'looking down' generationally speaking, people do not have a strong sense of lineage, and this view is in part governed by notions of good parenting, which tend to extend only one generation down. Grandchildren are generally viewed as the responsibility of one's own children, although as we have shown, specific relationships may be recognised (Finch 1996). So, while the specificity of relationships broadens, unpredictably, the scope of 'my family', the version of kinship that becomes embedded in the present through inheritance – although constituted in and about time – does not travel so far, temporally speaking.

Conclusion

What can we conclude about the nature of English kinship from our study of inheritance? We have argued that English kinship should be viewed primarily as a set of practices that are flexible and variable, with no rigid or fixed structure. In a sense, therefore, our data support ideas about the 'individualistic' nature of English kinship developed by Macfarlane and Strathern, which we introduced in Chapter 1. Macfarlane's version of individualism in kinship has the individual at the centre of his or her kin universe creating, more than joining, a family.

However, there are two misreadings of kinship that can result from a strong reliance on the concept of individualism. The first is the vision of an individual 'prime mover' at the centre of it all, who constructs their own biography as a 'reflexive project of the self' (Giddens 1991; 1992). Yet this version of individualistic practice is entirely at odds with our data, which consistently point to relational practices, whether they involve the use of inherited money, the constitution of keepsakes, or whatever. The second is the tendency for the concept of individualism to imply a rather static argument in which an individual 'selects' the composition of his or her family for all time. Our discussion of the significance of time for kinship and inheritance demonstrates that we need to conceptualise kinship as relational in order to see how it is a way of organising time. The significance of time is lost if we construe kinship to mean 'the family' of an 'individual'.

We have presented a strong case for an understanding of English kinship that emphasises its relational more than individual nature. It is fundamentally the relationships between people, in a dynamic sense, that constitute kinship and make it 'work'. The debate we charted in Chapter 1 about whether English kinship is best characterised as based on persons or positions essentially misses the point. English kinship is based on *relations*.

The principle of testamentary freedom in English law is highly supportive of this flexible kind of kinship, because essentially it privileges the right of testators to decide how to dispose of their property, possessions and assets. It therefore gives a high degree of flexibility to those who choose to make wills, whatever their personal vision of 'my inheritance family'. For those who do not, English intestacy provisions produce a much more constrained and fixed version of kinship, where spouse, biological children and 'full' blood kin have priority as beneficiaries, and which is underpinned by notions of hetero-normativity (Finch *et al.* 1996). Where testamentary freedom makes no assumptions about appropriate structures and hierarchies of relationships, intestacy provisions produce a very clear version that may be at odds with what people want to do and with the ways in which they live their family relationships. This makes it imperative for those who wish to construct a version of their 'inheritance family' that differs from the intestacy version to make a will, a point emphasised by many of the solicitors we interviewed.

The flexibility of English kinship is highly valued, and it permits reformulation and adaptation to social and demographic change. Our analysis of families with experience of divorce, separation, repartnering and step-relationships in Chapter 2 points to the dynamic ways in which English kinship is being refashioned by people in changing contexts. It also points to the importance of the principle of testamentary freedom in underpinning these relationships for inheritance purposes. This suggests that English kinship has a rather distinctive character, centring on a flexibility that people hold dear. Even where inheritance 'choices' look predictable, for example when a spouse inherits all or when children get equal shares, we must not underestimate the significance of the fact that these patterns emerge through processes of *negotiation*, not *regulation*. Nowhere in our data is there any suggestion that people would like a tighter framework, or less choice, in how they activate kinship in their inheritance practices. On the contrary, in this context it seems that the principle of testamentary freedom is to be highly prized. Any moves to limit its scope and to curtail the flexibility and negotiated character of kin relationships would be fundamentally out of step with how people make English kinship work.

Appendix A
Methodology

The 'inheritance project' was made up of three linked empirical studies: a study of 800 wills; a study of eighty-eight interviews with ninety-eight individuals; and a study of interviews with thirty solicitors and wills advisers.

The wills study

The wills study drew on data from 800 probated wills. Full details of the methodology and analytical framework for this study are given in *Wills, Inheritance and Families* (Finch *et al.* 1996), where the detailed analysis of that data set is presented. We used the wills to trace patterns of bequeathing and the family and non-family relationships that people recognise in wills.

The wills were sampled randomly from probate calendars held at Somerset House. Prior to making our selections, we stratified our sample in two ways: by year and by region. We sampled 200 from each of the years 1959, 1969, 1979 and 1989. The purpose of this was to allow us to investigate whether there had been clear changes in patterns of bequeathing over the period when home ownership has spread rapidly. Information about the testator's address at the time of death enabled us to stratify the sample by region. Half our sample were wills of people who had died in the south-east of England and half in the north-west. Our reason for building in this regional comparison was to ensure that we would pick up any variation in patterns of bequeathing consequent upon the higher value of houses in the south-east.

In the course of our analysis we constructed variables from the information available to us. The probate calendars enabled us to identify a range of testator characteristics: gender, region, estate size and date of death. However, we should point out here that our random sample was based on the year in which wills were probated, not the dates when they were written. This information was available to us in the will but was not indicated in the probate calendars from which our random sample was drawn. In addition, we constructed a variable for marital status (which has some limitations, discussed in Finch *et al.* 1996). We were not able to construct variables for ethnicity or social class because of inadequate information.

We used these variables to analyse patterns of bequeathing identified in the wills, using a range of measures. These included analysis of the overall patterns of first-choice beneficiaries and bequests; details of first-substitute beneficiaries and bequests; details of beneficiaries and bequests featured at the second and subsequent levels of substitution; information on each individual beneficiary; and details of people mentioned in the will who did not receive a bequest. Our analysis was undertaken using SPSSX version 4.

The interview study

The aim of the interview study was to discover how inheritance is handled in 'ordinary families'. We wanted to discover how people negotiated inheritance with their kin. In using the term 'ordinary families', we meant to convey that our focus was specifically *not* upon aristocratic or wealthy families, or those who had held land or considerable property over many generations.

Our sampling strategy was guided by theoretical principles that we have used in previous work (Finch and Mason 1990b). Our aim was to generate a study group that would include a theoretically meaningful range of interviewee characteristics and experiences. These would allow us to make comparisons, enabling us to develop and test out our interpretations and analyses using theoretical principles. As we have done before, we used the logic of analytic induction in the analytical process. This involves the systematic search for 'negative instances' and alternative explanations across a range of relevant situations (Denzin 1989; Mason 1996b).

Thus our study group is not intended to be representative of the wider population in an empirical sense. Indeed, it would be impossible to produce a representative sample of 'kin groups', given our arguments about the fluid and relational nature of kinship. Instead, our study group allows us to bring into play characteristics and experiences that are especially pertinent for inheritance and kinship, and to make meaningful comparisons on which we build our more general arguments.

We set out below the key interviewee characteristics and experiences that we built into our study group of ninety-eight interviewees. As the study population size is so close to 100, we use real numbers rather than percentages for the most part.

- *Gender*. We wanted a reasonably even split so that we had enough cases to explore variation within as well as across gender categories. Our final study group included fifty-eight women and forty men.
- *Housing tenure*. We wanted to include significant numbers of home owners because of the possible links that we have discussed between home ownership and patterns of inheritance. Additionally, we felt it important to include people who were the first generation in their families to own a home. We were interested to know whether the 'newness' (generationally speaking) of the experience of owning property might give people a distinctive perspective on matters of inheritance and kinship. We also wanted people with other forms of housing tenure so that we could make meaningful comparisons. Our final study group included seventy-five owner-occupiers, twenty-two (29 per cent) of whom were first-generation home owners; thirteen people in rented accommodation; and ten who were living in the family home.
- *Divorce, separation, repartnering and step-relationships*. We anticipated that these experiences might raise complex issues in relation to inheritance and kinship. Forty-six of the interviewees (twenty-nine women and seventeen men) in our study had such experiences either personally or in their close family. In terms of current marital status, sixty were married (roughly equal numbers of men and women); five were divorced (all women); five were remarried (all but one were women); nine were widowed (all but one were women); fifteen were single (five women, ten men); and five were cohabiting (three women and two men).
- *Age*. We wanted a range of ages, but we reasoned that matters of inheritance might be more of a 'live issue' for older rather

than younger cohorts, so we skewed our study group towards middle-aged and older people. The ages of interviewees in our final study group ranged from 18 to 89. Twenty-four were under 40, thirty-two were in their forties, fifteen in their fifties and twenty-seven over 60.

- *Ethnicity.* Although we have not designed a study to probe the significance of ethnic diversity in all its variations, we wanted to make sure that our study group was not simply based on the white English experience. We aimed to include some interviewees of other ethnic origins, of Asian descent in particular. Our final study group included fifteen people of Asian origin (seven women and eight men), and two (both women) who were white British married to someone of Asian origin. The rest were of white British descent.
- *People for whom paying for care had been an issue.* We anticipated that deliberations about paying for care might raise important questions about property ownership between generations. Thirty-four (twenty-one women and thirteen men) interviewees reported to us that this had been a live issue for them or for a close relative.
- *Wills.* We wanted to ensure that we included people who had made wills as well as those who had not. Forty people in our study population had made a will, and fifty-eight had not.
- *Experience of being a beneficiary.* Again, we wanted to include some people who had had this experience. Interviewees in our study reported a total of 102 examples of receiving an inheritance (some had inherited more than once).
- *Kin groups.* Here we would interview more than one member of a family so that we could gain access to different perspectives on similar issues from within the same family grouping. Our final study group included thirty-two people who were in the study population as individuals, twenty who were in the study population as part of a couple or 'pair' of relatives, and forty-six who were in the study as part of a 'kin group' where we interviewed between three and eight relatives.

We gained our study group through a variety of mechanisms, including drawing names and addresses from the electoral register and targeting specific geographical areas known to contain certain forms of housing and tenure. We also contacted residential care homes and sheltered housing schemes to gain access to older interviewees and, in order to inflate our sample of interviewees of Asian descent where we had particular difficulties in gaining access to respondents, we used personal contacts.

Almost all the interviews were conducted by Lynn Hayes and Lorraine Wallis during 1991 and 1992. The interviews were semi-structured and designed in such a way that the interviewers could follow up specific examples of inheritance and related practices with each interviewee in a way sensitive to their own biographies. All interviews were tape-recorded (where the interviewees agreed) and fully transcribed. The data were analysed in various ways, including the use of NUD*IST, the qualitative data analysis software package.

All interviewees are referred to by pseudonyms throughout. Where we quote directly from our transcripts, we include brief details about the interviewee: their pseudonym, their age group, and their marital and tenure status.

The solicitors study

Our small study of solicitors was exploratory. Our aim was to discover the perspectives of wills advisers and solicitors on the process and practice of making a will and its relationship to kinship. Specifically, we were interested in their role in the processes of will making and probate, and their views on the ways in which family relationships are recognised and dealt with within these (further findings from the solicitors study and details of its methodology can be found in Masson 1994a; 1994b).

We interviewed thirty solicitors and wills advisers, and these interviews were undertaken by Janet Finch, Jennifer Mason and Judith Masson during 1992 and 1993. The interviewees were located in towns in the Midlands or the north of England. Four of the interviewees worked for the major banks or their associated trust departments. The other twenty-six worked for firms of solicitors. We selected our study group to include firms ranging in age and size. The smallest was a sole practitioner (one interviewee), and the largest involved firms with ten or more partners (four interviewees). We selected solicitors across a range of city centre and suburban practices. Our study group included seven women and twenty-three men. Three of the interviewees were of Asian origin (all men) working in practices largely serving Asian communities.

We arranged our interviews by telephoning each firm and asking for the name of the person who dealt with wills and probate. We then contacted that person and arranged a meeting for a half-hour interview (although some lasted considerably longer at the interviewee's instigation). We had no refusals. Our interviews were semi-structured, and the data were written up into interview notes, which were analysed in a variety of ways, including use of NUD*IST.

Bibliography

Adam, B. (1990) *Time and Social Theory*, Cambridge: Polity Press.
Allan, G. (1979) *A Sociology of Friendship and Kinship*, London: Allen & Unwin.
Aries, P. (1983) *The Hour of Our Death*, London: Allen & Unwin.
Bauman, Z. (1988) *Freedom*, Milton Keynes: Open University Press.
—— (1992) *Postmodern Ethics*, Oxford: Blackwell.
—— (1995) *Life in Fragments*, Oxford: Blackwell.
Beck, U. (1992) *Risk Society: Towards a New Modernity*, New York: Sage.
Beck, U. and Beck-Gernsheim, E. (1995) *The Normal Chaos of Love*, Cambridge: Polity Press.
Benhabib, S. (1992) *Situating the Self: Gender, Community and Postmodernism within Contemporary Ethics*, Bloomington: Indiana University Press.
Berking, H. (1999) *Sociology of Giving*, London: Sage.
Brannen, J. (1999) 'Children's family networks and significant others', unpublished paper presented to the ESRC Seminar Group on 'Postmodern Kinship', University of Leeds.
Cheal, D. (1988) *The Gift Economy*, London: Routledge.
Davey, J. A. (1996a) *Equity Release: An Option for Older Home Owners*, University of York: Centre for Housing Policy Research report.
—— (1996b) 'Equity release for older home owners', in *Findings*, York: Joseph Rowntree Foundation.
Delphy, C. and Leonard, D. (1992) *Familiar Exploitation*, Cambridge: Polity Press.
Denzin, N. K. (1989) *The Research Act: A Theoretical Introduction to Sociological Methods* (third edition), Englewood Cliffs, NJ: Prentice Hall.
Edwards, J., Franklin, S., Hirsch, E., Price, F. and Strathern, M. (1993) *Technologies of Procreation: Kinship in the Age of Assisted Conception*, Manchester: Manchester University Press.

Finch, J. (1987) 'Kinship and friendship', in Jowell, R., Witherspoon, S. and Brook, L. (eds) *British Social Attitudes: Special International Report*, Aldershot: Gower.
—— (1989) *Family Obligations and Social Change*, Cambridge: Polity Press.
—— (1996) 'Inheritance and financial transfers in families', in Walker, A. (ed.) *The New Generational Contract: Intergenerational Relations, Old Age and Welfare*, London: UCL Press.
Finch, J. and Hayes, L. (1994) 'Inheritance, death and the concept of home' *Sociology* Vol. 28, No. 2: 417–34.
—— (1995) 'Gender, inheritance and women as testators', in Lyon, S. and Morris, L. (eds) *Gender Relations in Public and Private: Changing Research Perspectives*, London: Macmillan.
Finch, J. and Mason, J. (1990a) 'Filial obligations and kin support for elderly people', *Ageing and Society* Vol. 10: 151–75.
—— (1990b) 'Decision taking in the fieldwork process: theoretical sampling and collaborative working', in Burgess, R. G. (ed.) *Studies in Qualitative Methodology*, Vol. 2, London: JAI Press, 25–50.
—— (1991) 'Obligations of kinship in contemporary Britain: is there normative agreement?' *British Journal of Sociology* Vol. 42, No. 3: 349–67.
—— (1993) *Negotiating Family Responsibilities*, London: Routledge.
Finch, J. and Wallis, L. (1993) 'Death, inheritance and the life course', in Clark, D. (ed.) *The Sociology of Death: Sociological Review Monograph*, Oxford: Blackwell, 50–68.
Finch, J., Mason, J., Masson, J., Hayes, L. and Wallis, L. (1996) *Wills, Inheritance and Families*, Oxford: Oxford University Press.
Firth, R., Hubert, J. and Forge, A. (1970) *Families and Their Relatives*, London: Routledge & Kegan Paul.
Flowerdew, J. (1999) 'Reformulating familiar concerns: parents in stepfamilies', University of Leeds: unpublished PhD thesis.
Forrest, R. and Murie, A. (1989) 'Differential accumulation: wealth, inheritance and housing policy', *Policy and Politics* Vol. 17, No. 2: 25–39.
—— (eds) (1995) *Housing and Family Wealth: Comparative International Perspectives*, London: Routledge.
Franklin, A. (1995) 'Family networks, reciprocity and housing wealth', in Forrest, R. and Murie, A. (eds) *Housing and Family Wealth: Comparative International Perspectives*, London: Routledge.
Giddens, A. (1991) *Modernity and Self Identity*, Cambridge: Polity Press.
—— (1992) *The Transformation of Intimacy*, Cambridge: Polity Press.
Goffman, E. (1972) *Interaction Ritual*, Harmondsworth: Penguin.
Goody, J. (1976) 'Introduction', in Goody, J., Thirsk, J. and Thompson, E. P. (eds) *Family and Inheritance: Rural Society in Western Europe 1200–1800*, Cambridge: Cambridge University Press.

Goody, J., Thirsk, J. and Thompson, E. P. (eds) (1976) *Family and Inheritance: Rural Society in Western Europe 1200–1800*, Cambridge: Cambridge University Press.

Goulbourne, H. (1999) 'The transnational character of Caribbean kinship in Britain', in McRae, S. (ed.) *Changing Britain: Families and Households in the 1990s*, Oxford: Oxford University Press.

Hamnett, C. (1991) 'A nation of inheritors? Housing inheritance, wealth and inequality in Britain', *Journal of Social Policy* Vol. 20: 509–36.

—— (1995) 'Housing inheritance and inequality: a response to Watt', *Journal of Social Policy* Vol. 24: 413–22.

—— (1996) 'Housing inheritance in Britain: its size, scale and future', in Walker, A. (ed.) *The New Generational Contract: Intergenerational Relations, Old Age and Welfare*, London: UCL Press.

Hamnett, C., Harmer, M. and Williams, P. (1991) *Safe as Houses: Housing Inheritance in Britain*, London: Paul Chapman.

Hekmann, S. J. (1995) *Moral Voices, Moral Selves: Carol Gilligan and Feminist Moral Theory*, Cambridge: Polity Press.

Jamieson, L. (1998) *Intimacy: Personal Relationships in Modern Societies*, Cambridge: Polity Press.

—— (1999) 'Intimacy transformed? A critical look at the "Pure Relationship" ', *Sociology* Vol. 33, No. 3: 477–94.

Macfarlane, A. (1978) *The Origins of English Individualism*, Oxford: Blackwell.

McGlone, F., Park, A. and Smith, K. (1998) *Families and Kinship*, London: Family Policy Studies Centre.

Mason, J. (1996a) 'Gender, care and sensibility in family and kin relationships', in Holland, J. and Adkins, L. (eds) *Sex, Sensibility and the Gendered Body*, Basingstoke: Macmillan.

—— (1996b) *Qualitative Researching*, London: Sage.

—— (2000) 'Deciding where to live: relational reasoning and narratives of the self', Centre for Research on Family, Kinship and Childhood, University of Leeds: Working Paper 19.

Masson, J. (1994a) 'Making wills, making clients (Part 1)', *The Conveyancer and Property Lawyer*, July–August: 267–74.

—— (1994b) 'Making wills, making clients (Part 2)', *The Conveyancer and Property Lawyer*, September–October: 360–9.

Mauss, M. (1954) *The Gift: Forms and Functions of Exchange in Archaic Societies*, London: Cohen & West.

Millar, J. and Warman, A. (1996) *Family Obligations in Europe*, London: Family Policy Studies Centre.

Morgan, D. H. J. (1976) *Social Theory and the Family*, London: Routledge.

—— (1996) *Family Connections*, Cambridge: Polity Press.

Munro, M. (1987) 'Housing, wealth and inheritance', *Journal of Social Policy* Vol. 17, No. 4: 417–36.

Office for National Statistics (1999) *Social Trends*, London: HMSO.

Schneider, D. M. (1968) *American Kinship: A Cultural Account*, Englewood Cliffs, NJ: Prentice Hall.

Scott, J. (1982) *The Upper Classes: Property and Privilege in Britain*, London: Macmillan.

Segalen, M. (1986) *Historical Anthropology of the Family*, Cambridge: Cambridge University Press.

Sevenhuijsen, S. (1998) *Citizenship and the Ethics of Care*, London: Routledge.

Smart, C. and Neale, B. (1999) *Family Fragments?* Cambridge: Polity Press.

Smith, R. M. (ed.) (1984) *Land, Kinship and Life Cycle*, Cambridge: Cambridge University Press.

Stone, L. (1977) *The Family, Sex and Marriage in England 1500–1800*, London: Weidenfeld & Nicolson.

Strathern, M. (1992) *After Nature: English Kinship in the Twentieth Century*, Cambridge: Cambridge University Press.

Vogler, C. and Pahl, J. (1994) 'Money, power and inequality in marriage', *Sociological Review* Vol. 42: 263–88.

Watt, P. (1993) 'Housing inheritance and inequality: a rejoinder to Chris Hamnett', *Journal of Social Policy* Vol. 22: 527–34.

—— (1996) 'Social stratification and housing mobility', *Sociology* Vol. 30, No. 3: 533–50.

Weeks, J., Heaphy, B. and Donovan, C. (1999) 'Families of choice: autonomy and mutuality in non-heterosexual relationships', in McRae, S. (ed.) *Changing Britain: Families and Households in the 1990s*, Oxford: Oxford University Press.

Weiner, A. B. (1992) *Inalienable Possessions: The Paradox of Keeping-While-Giving*, Berkeley and Los Angeles: University of California Press.

Index

active parenting 48–9, 59, 175
Adam, B. 178
administration of small estates 62
agreements between beneficiaries 65
ancestor-centred kinship 19, 163–4, 179
Aries, Philippe 16
Asian interviewees 92–3, 96
assisted conception 18

Bauman, Z. 8, 21
Beck, U. 8–9, 14, 16, 20–1
Beck-Gernsheim, E. 8–9, 14, 21
beneficiaries, differential treatment of 77
Berking, H. 88
bilateral kinship 10
blood line 131–2; *see also* lineage
'blowing it' 101–2

care in old age, paying for 115–19, 136–7
children: as beneficiaries 174; claims of 40, 72, 86, 175; inherited money spent on 105; right to inherit 133
civil code 72
commemorative spending 100, 103–4, 109–10, 169
common stake in property *see* family property

'complex families' 25–6, 57–61
conflict over division of property 82–5
contested wills 83
continuity over time, sense of 15–16, 160
couple relationships, changing nature of 6–7
cremation 16
cultural traditions, diversity of 6

Davey, J.A. 122
death as a private event 16
Delphy, C. 13, 20, 163
dependency relationships 80–1, 87
division of property 66–7, 76; *see also* conflict
divorce 6–7, 26, 28, 35–6, 65, 174; *see also* 'complex families'

economic dimension of inheritance 12, 166
economic ties acknowledged through inheritance 87, 93, 175
ego-centred kinship 19, 21, 59, 163
English context, distinctiveness of 10, 17–19, 164, 167, 179–80
equal treatment, principle of 42–3, 49–51, 57, 76–9, 87, 130, 163, 168, 175–6; breaches of 79–82, 85, 93–4

equality of outcome in inheritance 45, 51, 53, 93, 175
equity release schemes 114–15, 120–2, 130
expectations of inheritance 60, 110, 133, 171

'family', use of term 4
'family practices' 4, 164
family property 20, 30, 59–60, 87, 98–9, 107–8, 128, 161, 171–2; strong concept of 130–3; *see also* transgenerational ownership
family provision legislation 68
family relationships: changing nature of 7; children's role in construction of 175; 'concentric circles' model of 10–11, 19; construction of 7–8, 178–9; defined according to circumstances 58–9; 'domestic economy' version of 178; mutual support within 13–14; and social life 5, 8–9; time dimension in 14–16, 108–9, 173
female family identity 170
financial planning 136
France 20, 163
friendships 151–2

gender differences and patterns 59, 64, 70, 86–7, 91, 106–7, 135, 142, 146, 153–4, 160, 168–71
Giddens, A. 8–9, 21
gifts, exchange of 88
giving away money 91–5
good parenting 123–7, 133, 137–8, 174–9
Goody, Jack 3
grandchildren: bequests to 73–4, 82; relationships with grandparents 7; responsibility for 133, 179

heirlooms 149–51
hoarding 98, 106, 148

holding strategy 98
'home', ideas of 129–30
home ownership 1–2; first- and second-generation 127; impact of inheritance on 12–13
houses: left for children 54–6, 129; regarded as financial assets 89, 130

in-law relationships 151–2
inalienable possessions 15, 142
inalienable right of people to control their assets 115, 121–2, 136, 171, 176
individualism 17–22, 57, 137, 163–4, 179–80; intensification of 21
inequality and inheritance 12–13
Inland Revenue statistics 71
intentions of interviewees about their own bequests 74–5
interviews with family members and professionals 23
intestacy legislation 62–3, 68, 134, 180
investment of inherited money 95–100

jewellery 56–7, 75, 129, 140, 142, 152, 158–9, 168
joint ownership: between spouses 71, 169, 174; of inherited money 99, 104–6

keeping inherited money 95–6
keeping objects other than keepsakes 149–51
keepsakes 103–4, 108, 141–6, 152–4, 160–1, 163–6, 169, 172, 176; getting into the 'wrong' hands 156–9; lifetime transmission of 155–6; second transmission of 152–4; treasuring of 146–9, 154

late modernity 8, 14, 17, 20–2

Index

Leonard, D. 13, 20, 163
life experiences 167–8
lifetime transfers 62, 155–6
lineage 163–4, 179; *see also* blood line

Macfarlane, Alan 19–22, 137, 163, 179
Major, John 2, 133
'major gifts' 73
marriages 14; first and subsequent 37–9, 58–9; *see also* 'complex families'; divorce; remarriage; spouses
Marx, Karl 19
Mason, J. 22
Mauss, M. 88
memories: carried by keepsakes 142, 146, 159–60; looking after 172–3, 177; loss of 159; sharing of 16–17
memory: activation of 172, 177–8; concept of 166
methodology of study 183–8
money, inheritance of 89–91
moral reasoning and moral difficulties 85, 88–103, 108–10, 173
Morgan, D.H.J. 4, 7, 14, 16, 164

narrative device 30, 112, 165, 167
Neale, B. 4, 7
nephews, bequests to 74
next of kin 73–4
nieces, bequests to 74
'nuclear' family 7–8

old age, financing of 112–38, 169, 171
opportunity spending, legacies used for 100–1
owner-occupation *see* home ownership
ownership: meaning of 136; sense of 98

Papua New Guinea 15
parent–child relationships 59–60, 86, 123, 126, 175–6; *see also* active parenting; good parenting
'passing out of the family' 30–3, 37–40, 59–60, 102, 174
patrimony 20, 163–4
personal identities, construction of 8–9, 13–14, 17, 21, 106, 109–10, 160
personal items of property 54, 56–7, 75–6, 82, 86, 129, 159–61, 174; unauthorised taking of 84; *see also* heirlooms; keepsakes
personal nature of elderly people's assets 117, 131, 135–8
personal relationships: between testators and beneficiaries 33–4, 86; embodied in objects 152–4, 172; maintained through inheritance 13–15; specificity of 173–4, 177–9
property: concepts of 87; and kinship 19–20; physical preservation of 128–30; reasoning about and use of 127–8; types of 53–4

reckless spending of inheritances 100–3
redistribution after an inheritance 92–4
relationism 22, 59, 137, 164
remarriage 26, 28, 35–6, 174; *see also* 'complex families'
reproduction: of kinship 15; of the social system 3
residue of an estate 68–9
rights of testators *see* testamentary freedom
routine spending, legacies used for 100–1

Scott, John 12
selection process for inheritance 58–9, 160–1, 174

selfishness, perceptions of 105–9
sentimental value 141–2
sharing of inherited money 104–6
Smart, C. 4, 7
social welfare 117, 136
'special' character of inherited money 96–8, 101, 173
spending of inherited money 100–4
spouses, inheritance between 31, 35–6, 39, 60, 69–71, 86–7, 128
stakeholding 136
step-children 27, 33, 45–9, 175
Stone, L. 21–2
Strathern, Marilyn 18–19, 22, 179
symbolism: of elderly people's assets 122, 135; of inherited money 98, 109; of inherited objects 15–17; of personal possessions 57, 101, 139–40, 148, 156, 160–1; of practices associated with inheritance 169–71

testamentary freedom 3, 11, 19–20, 34, 36, 72–3, 85, 137, 180–1

testators: attempting to control use of legacies 97, 99; bequests seen as unjust 94–5; respect for intentions of 84, 92, 108–9
time: organisation of 178–80; passage of 14–16, 98, 108–9, 173; *see also* continuity over time
transgenerational ownership 20, 111, 118, 122, 126, 131–8 *passim*, 163, 171–2, 177–8
travel as a reason for making a will 65
trusteeship, sense of 107, 128, 131
trusts 128

wealth, distribution of 166
Weber, Max 19
Weiner, Annette 15–16, 142, 160
will-making 26, 28, 50, 62–4, 74–5, 134, 180; reasons for 64–5
wills: study of 23; 'total estate' and 'composite' types 68–9, 168–9

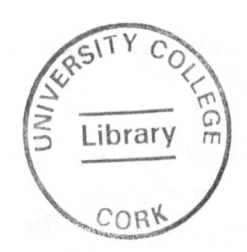

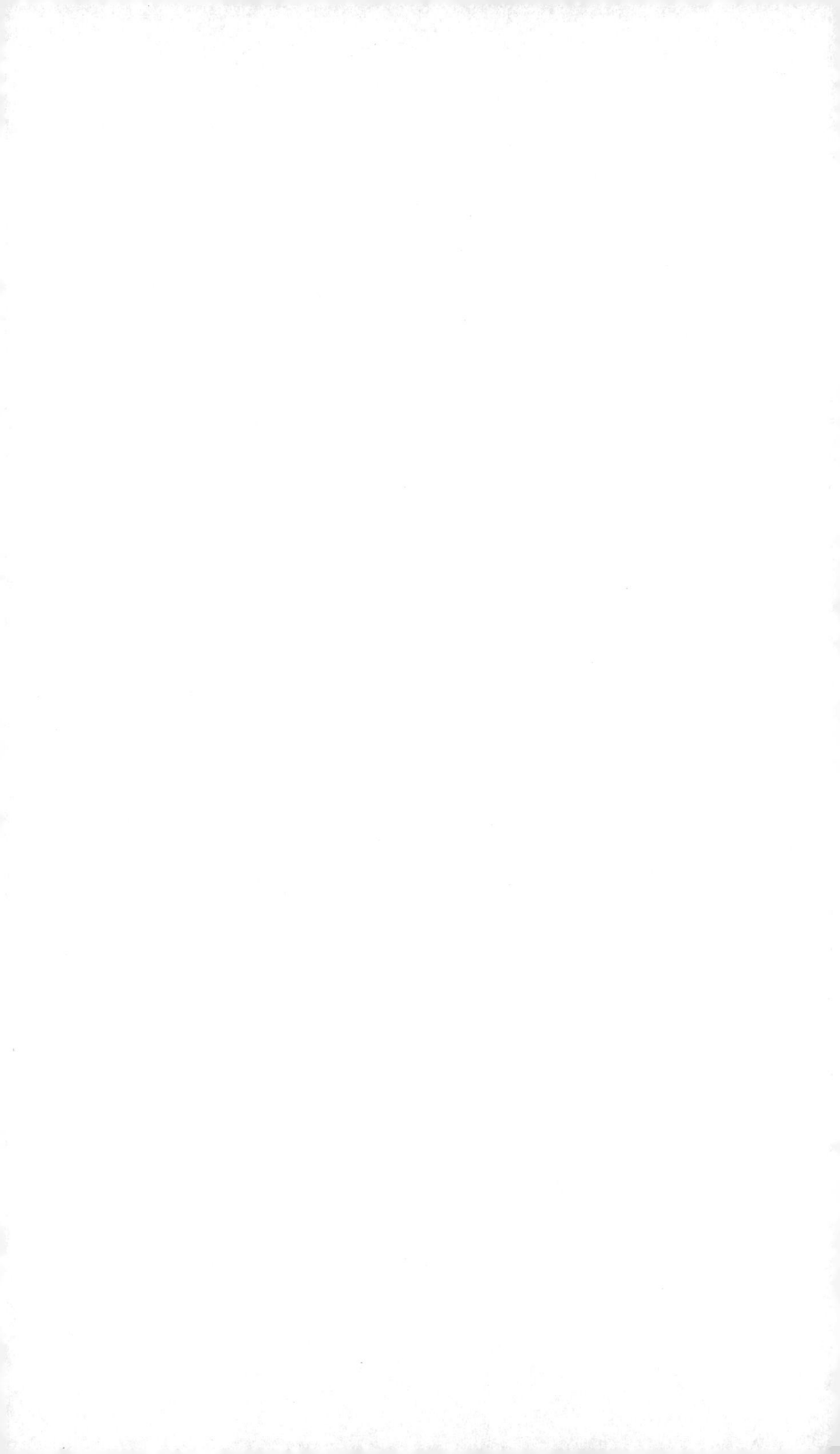